Lippincott's
Review Series

Community
and Home
Health
Nursing

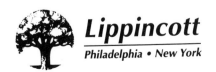

Lippincott

Philadelphia • New York

Lippincott's
Review Series

Community and Home Health Nursing

Judith A. Allender, RN C, MSN, EdD
Professor of Nursing
Department of Nursing
School of Health and Human Services
California State University
Fresno, California

Acquisitions Editor: **Susan M. Glover, RN, MSN**   Production Coordinator: **Adina LoBiondo**
Editorial Assistant: **Bridget Blatteau**   Design Coordinator: **Doug Smock**
Project Editor: **Barbara Ryalls**   Indexer: **Patricia Perrier**
Senior Production Manager: **Helen Ewan**

9 8 7 6 5 4 3 2 1

Library of Congress Cataloging-in-Publication Data

Allender, Judith Ann.
    Community and home health nursing / Judith A. Allender.
        p.   cm.—(Lippincott's review series)
    Includes bibliographical references and index.
    ISBN 0–397–55456–7 (alk. paper)
    1. Community health nursing—Examinations, questions, etc.
2. Home nursing—Examinations, questions, etc.   3. Community health
nursing—Outlines, syllabi, etc.   4. Home nursing—Outlines,
syllabi, etc.   I. Title.   II. Series.
    [DNLM: 1. Community Health Nursing—United States—examination
questions.   2. Home Care Services—United States—examination
questions.   3. Community Health Nursing—United States—outlines.
4. Home Care Services—United States—outlines.   WY 18.2 A432c
1997]
RT98.A47   1997
610.73′43′076—dc21
DNLM/DLC
for Library of Congress   97–19138
                                                                      CIP

Care has been taken to confirm the accuracy of the information presented and to describe generally accepted practices. However, the authors, editors, and publishers are not responsible for errors or omissions or for any consequences from application of the information in this book and make no warranty, express or implied, with respect to the contents of the publication.

The authors, editors and publisher have exerted every effort to ensure that drug selection and dosage set forth in this text are in accordance with current recommendations and practice at the time of publication. However, in view of ongoing research, changes in government regulations, and the constant flow of information relating to drug therapy and drug reactions, the reader is urged to check the package insert for each drug for any change in indications and dosage and for added warnings and precautions. This is particularly important when the recommended agent is a new or infrequently employed drug.

Some drugs and medical devices presented in this publication have Food and Drug Administration (FDA) clearance for limited use in restricted research settings. It is the responsibility of the health care provider to ascertain the FDA status of each drug or device planned for use in their clinical practice.

DEDICATION

To grandchildren—God's way of rewarding us for being parents—
especially Zachary, Kristin, Jeremy, Sydny, Nicolas, Nicole, Samuel, Ryan,
and Bence

REVIEWERS

Nellie C. Bailey, MS, MA, RN, CS
Associate Dean for Academic Programming/
Assistant Professor
State University of New York
Health Science Center at Brooklyn
College of Nursing
Brooklyn, New York

Harriet Rellis, RN, BSN, MSN, CRNP
Public Health Nurse IV, Nursing Supervisor
Bucks County Department of Health
Doylestown, Pennsylvania

INTRODUCTION

Lippincott's Review Series is designed to help you in your study of the key subject areas in nursing. The series consists of nine books, one in each core nursing subject area:

Community and Home Health Nursing
Critical Care Nursing
Fluids and Electrolytes
Maternal-Newborn Nursing
Medical-Surgical Nursing

Mental Health and Psychiatric Nursing
Pathophysiology
Pediatric Nursing
Pharmacology

Each book contains a comprehensive outlined content review plus chapter study questions and a comprehensive examination, both with, answer key with rationales for correct and incorrect responses.

Lippincott's Review Series was planned and developed in response to your request for outline review books that address each major subject area and also contain a self-test mechanism. These books meet the need for comprehensive subject review that will also assist you in identifying your strong and weak areas of knowledge. Each book is a complete source for review and self-assessment of a single core subject—all nine together provide an excellent comprehensive review of entry-level nursing.

Each book is all-inclusive of the content addressed in major textbooks. The content outline review uses a consistent nursing process format throughout and addresses nursing care for well and ill clients. Also included are necessary teaching and other concepts, including growth and development, nutrition, pharmacology, and body structures, functions and pathophysiology. Special features of each book are Key Concepts and Nursing Alerts, which are identified by distinctive icons. Key Concepts ☀ are basic facts the nurse needs to know to perform the job with ease and efficiency. Nursing Alerts ⚠ are fundamental guidelines the nurse can follow to ensure safe and effective care.

You can use the books in this series in several different ways. Overall, you can use them as subject reviews to augment general study throughout your basic nursing program and as a review to prepare for the National Council Licensure Examination (NCLEX-RN). How you use each book depends on your individual needs and preferences, and on whether you review each chapter systematically or concentrate only on those chapters whose subject areas are particularly problematic or challenging.

You may instead choose to use the comprehensive examination as a self-assessment opportunity to evaluate your knowledge base before you review the content outline. Likewise, you can use the study questions for pre- or post-testing after study, followed by the comprehensive examination as a means of evaluating your knowledge and competencies of an entire subject area.

Regardless of how you use the books, one of the strengths of the series is the self-assessment opportunity it offers in addition to guidance in studying and reviewing content. The chapter study questions and comprehensive examination questions have been carefully developed to cover all topics in the outline review. Most importantly, each question is categorized according to the components of the National Council of State Boards of Nursing Licensing examination (NCLEX).

▶ Cognitive Level: Knowledge, Comprehension, Application, or Analysis
▶ Client Need: Safe, Effective Care Environment (Safe Care); Physiological Integrity (Physiologic): Psychosocial Integrity (Psychosocial); and Health Promotion and Maintenance (Health Promotion)
▶ Phase of the Nursing Process: Assessment, Analysis (Dx), Planning, Implementation, Evaluation

For those questions not related to a client need or to a phase of the nursing process, NA (not applicable) will be used, as in questions that test knowledge of a basic science.

Unlike the NCLEX examination that tests the cumulative knowledge needed for safe practice by an entry-level nurse, these practice tests systematically evaluate the knowledge base that serves as the building block for the entire nursing educational process. In this way, you can prepare for the NCLEX examination throughout your course of study. Good study habits throughout your educational program are not only the best way to ensure ongoing success, but also will prove the most beneficial way to prepare for the licensing examination.

Keep in mind that these books are not intended to replace formal learning. They cannot substitute for textbook reading, discussion with instructors, or class attendance. Every effort has been made to provide accurate and current information, but class attendance and interaction with an instructor will provide invaluable information not found in books. Used correctly, these books will help you increase understanding, improve comprehension, evaluate strengths and weaknesses in areas of knowledge, increase productive study time, and, as a result, help you improve your grades.

MONEY BACK GUARANTEE—Lippincott's Review Series will help you study more effectively during coursework throughout your educational program, and help you prepare for quizzes and tests, including the NCLEX exam. If you buy and use any of the nine volumes in Lippincott's Review Series and fail the NCLEX exam, simply send us verification of your exam results and your copy of the review book to the address below. We will promptly send you a check for our suggested list price.

Lippincott's Review Series
Marketing Department
Lippincott-Raven Publishers
227 East Washington Square
Philadelphia, PA 19106-3780

ACKNOWLEDGMENTS

I would like to thank my editor Susan Glover for suggesting I develop this book, *Community and Home Health Nursing,* to be a part of **Lippincott's Review Series.** Her help and patience throughout its progress is appreciated. The insightful contributions of Deedie McMahon as a developmental editor on this project are also much appreciated. I also want to thank Galen Gattis, RN, MSN, for his research assistance that helped develop major parts of this book and the insightful editorial comments from Anita Solis, RN, Inservice Educator at BestCare Home Health Agency, Hanford, CA. It is our collective hope that through the use of this review book nursing students will be prepared to provide appropriate nursing care to clients in a variety of community settings and at home. It is a changing health care delivery system—a restructured system that demands the highest quality of nursing and health care be delivered in the most cost-effective manner. This brings the nurse to aggregates and to clients in their homes.

Judy

CONTENTS

Lippincott's
Review Series

Community
and Home
Health
Nursing

Review of Community Health Nursing

Unit I
Introduction to Community Health Nursing*

---

*Throughout this book the term community health can be used interchangeably with public health.

Health as Perceived
in the Community

I. Definitions of Health

A. World Health Organization: "a state of complete physical, mental, and social well-being and not merely the absence of disease or infirmity" (Pickett & Hanlon, 1990). This classic definition is idealistic and serves as a goal that is difficult, if not impossible, to reach.

B. Other
   1. "a state of equilibrium between humans and the physical, biologic, and social environment . . ." (Last, 1987)
   2. "a state of wellness which includes soundness of mind, body, and spirit" (Spradley & Allender, 1996)
   3. "fitness as a result of individual adaptation to stress" (Leahy, Cobb, & Jones, 1982)
   4. "an integrated method of functioning which is oriented toward maximizing the potential of which the individual is capable within the environment where he is functioning" (Dunn, 1961)

3

5. Wellness is a dynamic state, is influenced by internal and external variables, and each person, group, or community has the potential for growth.

II.   Definitions of Community Health

 A. Winslow (1920): "Public health is the science and art of preventing disease, prolonging life, and promoting health and efficiency through organized community efforts for the sanitation of the environment, the control of communicable infections, the education of the individual in personal hygiene, the organization of medical and nursing services for the early diagnosis and preventive treatment of disease, and the development of the social machinery to insure everyone a standard of living adequate for the maintenance of health, so organizing these benefits as to enable every citizen to realize his birthright of health and longevity." (Pickett & Hanlon, 1990, p. 5)

B. Other

1. "Community health is the identification of needs and the protection and improvement of collective health within a geographically defined area." (Spradley & Allender, 1996)

2. "Meeting collective needs by identifying problems and managing interactions within the community and larger society. The goal of community-oriented practice." (Stanhope & Lancaster, 1992)

III.   Basic Concepts

 A. The Wellness–Illness Continuum

1. A visual display of a person's level of health represented by a symbol on the continuum (Fig. 1-1)

2. The goal is to move closer to the wellness end of the continuum through individual, group, community, national, and worldwide efforts to improve personal and environmental health.

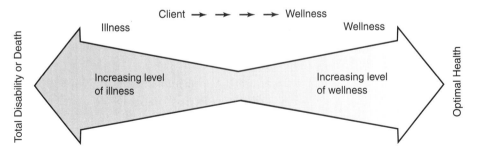

FIGURE 1-1.
The wellness–illness continuum. The level of illness increases as one moves toward disability or death; the level of wellness increases as one moves toward optimal health. This continuum shows the relative nature of health. At any given time a person can be placed at some point along the continuum.

B. **The Six Community Health Services**

1. *Promotion:* includes all efforts and services designed to move people closer to an optimal level of well-being or to higher levels of wellness

    a. Increase span of a healthy life for all people
    b. Reduce disparities in health among population groups
    c. Offer preventive services for all people

2. *Prevention:* anticipates and averts problems or discovers them as early as possible to minimize possible disability and impairment

    a. **Primary (health teaching and preventing illnesses or injuries from occurring)**
    b. **Secondary (early diagnosis and treatment or intervention)**
    c. **Tertiary (initiated to minimize disability and help restore function in existing health problems; Display 1-1)**

3. *Treatment*

    a. Focuses on the illness end of the wellness–illness continuum
    b. Provides direct services to people with health problems (eg, a neighborhood health center that provides health screening, education, and referral services)
    c. Offers indirect services that help people obtain treatment (eg, the advocacy role of all health team members and information and referral services)
    d. Develops programs to correct unhealthy conditions (eg, initiate a substance abuse treatment center, develop new regulations to eliminate water pollution in a community lake)

4. *Rehabilitation:* seeks to reduce disability and, if possible, restore function

    a. Individuals (eg, physical and occupational therapy for people with chronic and debilitative disease, and for an aging population [rehabilitative and long-term services])
    b. Groups and communities (eg, groups such as Alcoholics Anonymous, ostomy clubs, or the creation of a park in a vacant inner city lot)

DISPLAY 1-1.
Examples of the Three Levels of Prevention

Primary prevention—health teaching (eg, diet, rest, exercise, sleep needs, safety), immunizations
Secondary prevention—screening procedures, (eg, TB skin tests, self-breast exams [SBE], and self-testicular exams [STE])
Tertiary prevention—rehabilitation (eg, teaching breathing techniques to a COPD client, exercise regimen post-hip fracture, medication compliance follow-up for a client with TB classification III diagnosis)

      5. *Evaluation:* analyzes, judges, evaluates, and improves community health practice according to established goals and standards

         a. Individual: Are client outcomes being reached?

         b. Program: Are goals meeting the needs of the target population?

      6. *Research:* systematically explores the effects of community health and practice through scientific investigations and epidemiology (see Chaps. 7 and 11).

IV. Client Focus

A. *Populations:* **groups of people who share one or more environmental or personal characteristic. Community health is primarily focused on populations and moves beyond the provision of direct care to individuals and families.**

    1. Concerned with distinct and overlapping subpopulations (eg, teenagers, teenagers who are pregnant, teenagers in gangs, pregnant teenagers in gangs)

    2. Provided to those who seek out health services as well as for those who do not

B. *Aggregates:* **group of people who share some common interest, goal, or problem**

    1. Considered a unified whole when solving problems or promoting health

    2. Frequently receive care in community health practice (the students in a school, elderly in a senior center, workers in a factory, families in a housing development)

    3. **Services determined by a needs assessment, collaborative plan, implementation, and scientific evaluation**

C. *Families:* **a group of people integrated, interacting, and interdependent. Families may be the unit of service in the community because of certain high-risk behaviors or for individualized caregiving that focuses on family growth, health promotion, or health maintenance.**

    1. High-risk lifestyle behaviors that jeopardize individual health

    2. Chronic illnesses

    3. Communicable diseases

    4. Environmental issues needing investigation and/or resolution

D. *Individuals:* **one member of a family or a group. Although the individual may be the focus of care, his/her level of health influences others, and affects the extent of nursing care.**

V. Community Health Nursing

  A. Definitions

    1. The branch or specialty of nursing that focuses on the interrelatedness of health conditions, illness prevention and health

promotion in aggregates in the community and in particular vulnerable populations (Spradley & Allender, 1996)

2. The field of nursing that synthesizes the public health sciences and the theory of nursing to improve the health of individuals, families, and communities (Stanhope & Lancaster, 1992)

3. "Public health nursing may be defined as a field of professional practice in nursing and in public health in which technical nursing, interpersonal, analytical, and organizational skills are applied to problems of health as they affect the community. These skills are applied in concert with those of other persons engaged in health care, through comprehensive nursing care of families and other groups and through measures for evaluation of the public, and for mobilization of the public for health action." (Freeman, 1963).

 4. **"Public health nursing synthesizes the body of knowledge from the public health sciences and professional nursing theories for the purpose of improving the health of the entire community. This goal lies at the heart of primary prevention and health promotion and is the foundation for public health nursing practice. To accomplish this goal, public health nurses work with groups, families, and individuals as well as in multidisciplinary teams and programs. Identifying subgroups (aggregates) within the population which are at high risk of illness, disability, or premature death, and directing resources toward these groups is the most effective approach for accomplishing the goal of public health nursing. Success in reducing the risks and in improving the health of the community depends on the involvement of consumers, especially groups experiencing health risks, and others in the community, in health planning, and in self-help activities." (American Public Health Association, 1981)**

5. **"Community health nursing is a synthesis of nursing practice and public health practice applied to promoting and preserving the health of populations. The practice is general and comprehensive. It is not limited to a particular age group or diagnosis and is continuing, not episodic. The dominant responsibility is to the population as a whole; nursing directed to individuals, families, or groups contributes to the health of the total population. Health promotion, health maintenance, health education and management, coordination, and continuity of care are utilized in a holistic approach to the management of the health care of individuals, families, and groups in a community." (American Nurses Association, 1980)**

B. **Roles**

  1. *Clinician:* **provides health services to individuals, families, groups, and populations with a distinct difference from basic nursing**
      a. Holism: considers a broad range of interacting needs that affect the collective health of the "client" as a larger system (eg, a pregnant single mother with several children, who uses drugs, is alienated from her family, and has no permanent housing. The community health nurse's care goes far beyond a focus on labor and delivery)
      b. Wellness: focuses on health promotion and the prevention of illness, especially in high-risk groups and those interested in achieving a higher level of wellness
      c. Expansion of nursing skills: involves skills, such as observation, assessment, listening, communication, counseling, environmental awareness, collaboration, epidemiology and biostatistics, research, program evaluation, administration, leadership, and being an effective change agent
  2. *Educator:* **shares information formally (in larger groups as an invited speaker) and informally (with individuals, families and small groups based on need)**
      a. Directed toward clients in the community who are not acutely ill, and are better able to absorb and act on health information
      b. Valued because reaches a wider audience in the community
  3. *Advocate:* **acts on behalf of clients to help them achieve their rights, plead their cause, understand expected services, and partake in a complex health care delivery system. Nursing skills include:**
      a. Assertiveness
      b. Communication and negotiation
      c. Identification of resources and the ability to aquire them
  4. *Manager:* **exercises administrative direction toward the accomplishment of specified goals by using steps in the management process:**
      a. Planning—sets the goals and direction for the project and determines the means for achieving them
      b. Organizing—provides the structure in which people work
      c. Leading—works with people who need direction
      d. Controlling and evaluating—monitors and evaluates the effectiveness of the plan

    5. *Collaborator:* works jointly with others in a common en-
        deavor and cooperate as partners. Success depends on mul-
        tiprofessional and interdisciplinary collegiality
    6. *Leader:* directs, influences, or persuades others to effect
        change that will positively affect the health of clients (indi-
        viduals, families, groups, and communities)
    7. *Researcher:* engages in systematic investigation, collection,
        and analysis of data for the purpose of solving problems
        and, ultimately, enhancing community health practice
  C. Standards (Display 1-2)
  D. Influences
     1. On society
         a. The value of services provided by the community
             health nurse is often overlooked or unrecognized in
             the acute health care arena.
         b. Community health nurses serve clients on the "front
             line," often working with scant resources and provid-
             ing a service provided by few others.
         c. Society benefits when the population is healthy and
             productive.

DISPLAY 1-2.
Standards of Community Health Nursing Practice

Standard I—Theory. The nurse applies theoretical concepts as a basis for decisions in practice.

Standard II—Data Collection. The nurse systematically collects data that are comprehensive and accurate.

Standard III—Diagnosis. The nurse analyzes data collected about the community, family, and individual
to determine diagnoses.

Standard IV—Planning. At each level of prevention, the nurse develops plans that specify nursing actions
unique to client needs.

Standard V—Intervention. The nurse, guided by the plan, intervenes to promote, maintain, or restore
health, to prevent illness, and to effect rehabilitation.

Standard VI—Evaluation. The nurse evaluates responses of the community, family, and individual to interventions to determine progress toward goal achievement and to revise the data base, diagnoses, and
plan.

Standard VII—Quality Assurance and Professional Development. The nurse participates in peer review
and other means of evaluation to ensure quality of nursing practice. The nurse assumes responsibility
for professional development and contributes to the professional growth of others.

Standard VIII—Interdisciplinary Collaboration. The nurse collaborates with other health care providers,
professionals, and community representatives in assessing, planning, implementing, and evaluating
programs for community health.

Standard IX—Research. The nurse contributes to theory and practice in community health nursing through
research.

1986—American Nurses Association

   2. On health care organizations
       a. Organizations benefit by the expertise of the compre-
           hensive view of health care delivery the community
           health nurse brings to the setting.
       b. A primary prevention focus of the community health
           nurse helps the organization minimize health care
           costs.
       c. Health care services provided to clients in their homes,
           schools, and place of employment promote continuity
           of care, which is cost-effective and preferred by clients.
       d. Elimination or postponement of the need for admis-
           sion to acute care facilities is cost saving to health care
           organizations.
   3. On individual health
       a. Services keep individuals at a higher level of wellness,
           eliminating or postponing the need for admission to
           acute care settings.
       b. Individuals remain healthier when they have the skills
           necessary to meet their own health care needs.

VI. Dimensions

A. Practice Settings

   1. Homes: The traditional practice of visiting clients in the home
       continues and is the fastest growing sector of the health care
       system. Clients discharged from acute care settings frequently
       need follow-up care. The one-on-one care given in the home is
       an expensive, yet valuable service.
       a. Observation: visit clients in a comfortable setting and as-
           sess how they interact in their unique environment
       b. Accessibility: interact with clients who do not use health
           services regularly
       c. Knowledge deficit: assess clients' knowledge, actions, and
           resources, and increase their awareness of real or potential
           health problems
   2. Ambulatory settings: places that provide day or evening care,
       excluding overnight services

       a. Cost: reduces the cost of care for both the client and
           the health care delivery system, by providing care in
           clinics, outpatient departments of acute care facilities,
           a health maintenance organization (HMO), compre-
           hensive or single service neighborhood clinics, or day
           care centers
       b. Accessibility: physically and financially more accessible
           than acute care facilities. Services may not disrupt the
           clients' routine and allows them to return home faster.

3. Schools: public and private schools at all levels (preschool through college). The special skills and contributions of the community health nurse include health education, collaboration, and client advocacy. The nurse may be hired by the school district or contracted through a local health department.

   a. **Attendance: ensures that students attend classes in as healthy a state as possible without disabling or infectious processes that will hinder their learning or the learning of others**

   b. Accessibility: provides health education, health counseling, referrals and emergency care to students, as needed, throughout the day

4. Occupational settings (business/industry): contributes to the quality of individual lives, the productivity of business, and the well-being of the entire nation

   a. **Productivity: employees are hired to provide a service or to develop/produce a product. Health care increases the productivity of employees, which reduces product cost for consumers. In addition, negative work output is reduced.**

   b. Accessibility: provides health education, health counseling, referrals and emergency care to employees, as needed, in the workplace. Employees receive health care services without leaving the work setting, thus decreasing time away from the job.

5. Residential institutions: settings where clients reside in groups, either transitional (eg, halfway houses and rehabilitation centers) or long-term (eg, skilled nursing centers, assisted living centers, independent living centers for elders, and residential care centers)

   a. Cost: focuses on primary prevention and reduces care needed at the more expensive secondary or tertiary levels

   b. Accessibility: considers the ability level, safety and/or security needs of the client, and readily assesses, plans, and provides services for them

6. Correctional facilities: a large (and growing) group of clients with extensive health care needs, some resulting from their incarceration

   a. Safety and security: the first priorities of correctional facilities, not the health of individuals. However, health care services cannot be denied. A bevy of health care services are provided in correctional facilities at all three levels of prevention. Providing health care services within the facility protects clients, employees, and the larger community.

b. Cost: focuses on primary prevention in the facility, because transporting clients to health care services at the secondary or tertiary level of care is costly

B. Emerging Practice Settings

1. Homeless shelters: the numbers of homeless are increasing, primarily women and children. This increase demands new shelters with not only comprehensive nursing care, but also additional services (eg, three meals a day, showering and laundry facilities, day care and nap rooms for children, and work skill classes).

2. "On the street": services reach clients "on the street" in innovative ways.

   a. Gangs: active in many urban communities and are a new group community health nurses serve

   b. Clients with tuberculosis (TB): receive directly observed therapy (DOT). The community health nurse regularly administers medications to clients in bars, sleeping rooms, or at the client's "place" in a park. Note that most clients with TB do not live on the street.

   c. Substance abusers: receive informal counseling, health care services, and much needed referrals "on the street"

Bibliography

American Nurses Association (1980). *A conceptual model of community health nursing.* ANA Publication No. CH-10. Kansas City, MO: Author.

American Nurses Association (1986). *Standards of community health nursing practice.* Kansas City, MO: Author.

American Public Health Association (1981). *The definition and role of public health nursing in the delivery of health care.* Kansas City, MO: Author.

Dunn, H. (1961). *High level wellness.* Washington, DC: Mount Vernon Publishing.

Freeman, R. B. (1963). *Public health nursing practice.* (3rd ed.). Philadelphia: W. B. Saunders.

Last, J. M. (1987). *Public health and human ecology.* East Norwalk, CT: Appleton and Lange.

Leahy, K. M., Cobb, M. M., & Jones, M. C. (1982). *Community health nursing.* (4th ed.). New York: McGraw-Hill.

Pickett, G. E., & Hanlon, J. J. (1990). *Public health administration and practice.* (9th ed.). St. Louis: Times Mirror/Mosby.

Spradley, B. W., & Allender, J. A. (1996). *Community health nursing: Concepts and practice.* (4th ed.). Philadelphia: Lippincott-Raven.

Stanhope, M., & Lancaster, J. (1992). *Community health nursing: Process and practice for promoting health.* (3rd ed.). St. Louis: Mosby–Year Book.

STUDY QUESTIONS

1. The World Health Organization's definition of health includes:
   a. A state of complete physical, mental, and social well-being
   b. A state of equilibrium between humans and the environment
   c. Fitness as a result of individual adaptation to stress
   d. Soundness of mind, body, and spirit

2. The wellness–illness continuum is:
   a. A plan to promote the health of ill people
   b. A visual model of one's wellness or illness potential
   c. The implementation of health promotion activities
   d. The continual health and safety practices taught by nurses

3. An example of **primary prevention** is:
   a. Physical therapy for a knee injury
   b. Vision and hearing screening among school-age children
   c. TB skin tests for clinic employees
   d. Eating a well-balanced diet low in fat

4. An example of **secondary prevention** is:
   a. Physical therapy for a knee injury
   b. Vision and hearing screening among school-age children
   c. Participating in moderate exercise
   d. Eating a well-balanced diet low in fat

5. An example of **tertiary prevention** is:
   a. Physical therapy for a knee injury
   b. Vision and hearing screening among school-age children
   c. TB skin tests for clinic employees
   d. Eating a well-balanced diet low in fat

6. The primary focus of community health nursing is on:
   a. Individuals
   b. Families
   c. Groups
   d. Populations

7. Community health nursing services are provided to families in their homes when:
   a. An outpatient setting such as a clinic or doctor's office is closed
   b. The community health nurse has a lighter work schedule
   c. A disease or high-risk behavior may affect a family member's health
   d. There is a physician's order for a set of skilled nursing services

8. The American Nurses Association's (1980) definition of Community Health Nursing (CHN) includes the following concept:
   a. CHN is a speciality of nursing that works with vulnerable populations.
   b. CHN mobilizes the public for health action.
   c. The goal of CHN lies in primary prevention and health promotion.
   d. CHN is a synthesis of nursing practice and public health practice.

9. A community health nurse has many roles. One of the roles is providing holistic care with a wellness focus and involves expanding many basic nursing and caregiving skills. The role described above is:
   a. Educator
   b. Clinician
   c. Leader
   d. Collaborator

10. Practice settings for community health nurses vary. In one setting, the nurse may work with clients in outpatient departments of hospitals, through HMOs, or day care centers. These are examples of which of the following setting:
    a. Ambulatory settings
    b. Residential institutions
    c. Occupational health settings
    d. Correctional facilities

ANSWER KEY

1. *Correct response: a*
 b. This is from Last's (1987) definition of health.
 c. This is from Leahy, Cobb and Jones' definition of health (1982).
 d. This is part of the definition of health proposed by Spradley & Allender (1996).
Knowledge/NA/NA

2. *Correct response: b*
 Answer choices **a, c,** and **d** do not address that the wellness–illness continuum is a visual model to help depict where a person, group, or community is in regards to relative wellness or illness.
Knowledge/Health Promotion/ Assessment

3. *Correct response: d*
 a. Is an example of tertiary prevention.
 b. Is an example of secondary prevention.
 c. Is an example of secondary prevention.
Comprehension/Health Promotion/ Implementation

4. *Correct response: b*
 a. Is an example of tertiary prevention.
 c. Is an example of primary prevention.
 d. Is an example of primary prevention.
Comprehension/Health Promotion/ Implementation

5. *Correct response: a*
 b. Is an example of secondary prevention.
 c. Is an example of secondary prevention.
 d. Is an example of primary prevention.
Comprehension/Health Promotion/ Implementation

6. *Correct response: d*
 Answers **a, b,** and **c** are units of service, but the focus is on the health of large groups or populations that make up communities. At times, the health of one individual, family, or group may affect the health of the larger population, but the focus remains on the population level.
Knowledge/NA/NA

7. *Correct response: c*
 Answers **a** and **b**—home visits are not determined by office schedules or workload.
 Answer **d**—this describes Home Health Nursing Practice.
Comprehension/NA/Assessment

8. *Correct response: d*
 a. Is from the definition proposed by Spradley & Allender (1996).
 b. Is from the definition proposed by Freeman (1963).
 c. Is from the definition proposed by the American Public Health Association (1981).
Comprehension/NA/NA

9. *Correct response: b*
 a. The educator role focuses on health teaching.
 c. The leader role focuses on directing, influencing or persuading others.
 d. The collaborator role has the community health nurse working together with others as partners.
Application/NA/NA

10. *Correct response: a*
 b. Residential institutions are homelike settings where clients reside, usually in small groups.
 c. Occupational health settings include businesses and industries.
 d. In correctional facilities, the clients are ambulatory but are restricted to how and when they receive their health care.
Application/NA/NA

Global Historic Influences on Community Health and Community Health Nursing

I. Five Stages in the Disease History of Humankind (Polgar, 1964)

A. The Hunting and Gathering Era (before 10,000 BC)

1. For 2 million years, small groups of people (aggregates) wandered in search of food. Depending on their skill and availability, they ate a wide range of food, diverse in nutrients.

2. Aggregates suffered wounds from animals, other humans, and accidents; diseases from parasites, insect bites, and eating infected meat. Early death was common.

3. Contagious disease was uncommon because the aggregates were scattered, few in number, highly mobile, and never in contact with outside groups.

B.   **The Settled Village Era (10,000–6000 BC)**

1. The wandering groups eventually settled in small encampments, forming villages.
2. The concentration of people in small areas brought about different problems.
   a. Living close to animals caused diseases, such as salmonella, anthrax, Q fever, and tuberculosis (TB) in and among humans.
   b. Domestication of plants reduced the range of nutrients, compared with gathering foods, and possibly led to diseases of deficiency.
   c. The securing and ponding of water and removal of wastes caused diseases, such as typhus and typhoid, while mosquitoes spread malaria.

C.   **The Preindustrial Cities Era (6000 BC–1600 AD)**

1. As the population increased, villages became towns and cities.
2. Preexisting problems increased due to the larger number of animals and people living in a small area.
   a. Attempting to remove the increasing waste via the water supply led to increases in diseases, such as cholera.
   b. Rodent infestation facilitated the spread of plague.
   c. Diseases such as mumps, measles, influenza, and smallpox spread and became endemic due to the frequent contact among people living close together.
   d. At times, diseases became epidemic, spread by explorers and travelers; diseases such as syphilis became a challenge as a venereal disease.
   e. Occupational threats occurred as poisons were used in mining, metal processing, pottery making, fishing and hunting.

D.   **The Industrial Era (1600–1900 AD)**

1. Industrialization brought about dense and heavily populated urban areas.
2. Large cities attracted the poor, who hoped for a chance at "the good life." However, many problems affected people's health.
   a. Major problems included industrial waste, increased air and water pollution, and harsh working conditions.
   b. Common epidemics in the 1800s and 1900s were influenza, diphtheria, smallpox, typhoid fever, typhus, measles, malaria, and yellow fever.
   c. Exploration and imperialistic activities spread epidemics to populations with no immunity.

E.   **The Modern Era (1900–Present)**

1. Over the centuries, humans have attempted to adapt to sedentary living in overpopulated urban areas, with a place of living very different than that of our forefathers.

   2. Living in an industrialized society has not been without its problems. Death from communicable diseases has been replaced by other diseases. The following diseases have increased markedly in the past 100 years, especially in the last 50:
      a. Large bowel diseases, such as cancer, diverticulitis, and ulcerative colitis
      b. Venous disorders, including varicose veins, thrombosis, pulmonary embolism, and hemorrhoids
      c. Heart disease, diabetes, and gallstones
    3. Mortalities have changed in nature from infectious to chronic.
    4. Organized community efforts to prevent disease, prolong life, and promote health have occurred since prehistoric times.

II. The Evolution of Community Health Care Practices
   A. Early: health care practice based on superstition or sanitation; evolved as a way for many groups to survive

    1. Primitive societies, even before 6000 BC, used psychosomatic medicine (voodoo), isolation (banishment), and fumigation (smoke) to control disease and protect the clan or tribe.
   2. In each group there was a "healer" who administered a variety of therapeutic agents to the sick and injured.
   3. In Egypt and the Middle East, as early as 3000 BC, people built drainage systems, used toilets with water flushing systems, and practiced personal cleanliness.

   B. Biblical

    1. The Hebrew Hygienic Code: described in the Bible in Leviticus (1500 BC); emerged as the first written code and served as a model for personal and community sanitation

    2. Contributions of the Greeks and Romans
      a. Wealthy Greeks: emphasized personal hygiene, diet, and exercise, in addition to a sanitary environment (1000–400 BC)
      b. The Romans: developed laws regulating environmental sanitation, constructed paved streets, aqueducts, and a drainage system

   C. Middle Ages (500–1500 AD)
   1. Health care practices
      a. The decline of Rome (circa 500 AD): led to the Middle Ages; magic and religion used to treat health problems
      b. Physicians had little to offer; some public health measures considered, such as keeping wells and fountains clean and removing street refuse

      c.   Organized care occurred through monasteries; however, services were sporadic as monasteries became cloistered (not letting outsiders in)

     d.   The Crusaders: traveled across Europe and the Middle East, infecting many people with communicable diseases; contributed to the enlightenment that came in later centuries

  2. Major health care issues

     a.   Plague (Black Death): claimed one half of the world's population; led to the isolation, disinfection, and quarantine of ships; however, they were not to know why this helped for centuries

      b.   Leprosy: a classic disease that was handled by the church through isolation in leper houses, or leprosaria

      c.   Other communicable diseases: measles, smallpox, and diphtheria

D.   Renaissance (15th–17th centuries)

  1. Issues and responses

      a.   The Enlightenment: occurred due to trade expansion, population growth, and migration; interest in human dignity, human rights, and scientific truth

     b.   Elizabethan Poor Law (England, 1601): developed to deal with poverty; community (parishes) responsible for the care of the poor; governed for 200 years in England and became a prototype for later laws in the United States

  2. Leaders

      a.   (1546) Girolamo Fracastoro: presented a theory of infection as a cause and epidemic as a consequence of "seeds of disease"

      b.   (1567–1662) St Francis De Sales: developed a voluntary association of friendly visitors (with Madame de Chantal as director) to go to the homes of the poor and care for the sick

     c   (1576–1669) St. Vincent De Paul: organized the Sisterhood of the Dames de Charite, which introduced the modern and sound principles of visiting nursing and social welfare; aim was to help people help themselves

      d.   (1676) Anton van Leeuwenhoek: invented a microscope and described the organisms; however, he did not associate them with disease

E.   18th Century (The Industrial Revolution)

   1. **1750–1830: Influential in regard to the future design of community health services**

2. **Health problems: included a high infant mortality rate (at times the murder of illegitimate infants), poor and unsafe working conditions, occupational diseases, and a growing incidence of mental illness**
3. The mentally ill: until this time, they were committed to madhouses, jails, or workhouses. Major strides were taken (Vincenzo Chiarugi—1788) to establish a system in which properly trained nurses cared for the mentally ill in asylums, providing kindness, physical exercise, good food, and fresh air.
4. Growth of United States hospitals: paralleled the development of asylums. Many major hospitals on the East Coast have their roots back to the mid 1700s.

F. **Modern Medicine, Public Health and Nursing (1800s)**
  1. Medical science changes
     a. The "spontaneous generation" theory: before the 1800s, physicians believed that disease organisms grew from nothing. Treatment included bloodletting, starving, using leeches, and administering large doses of metals and antimony.

     b. **The germ theory: crowning achievement of the 19th century. Scientists used Leeuwenhoek's microscope to identify microbes as the causative factor in disease.**
  2. The development of organized public health
     a. America experienced unprecedented growth as Europeans poured into the United States. People began moving west, spreading diseases to new areas and territories. In addition, hospital care was inadequate.
     b. Health departments developed to protect the populations. The earliest was founded in Baltimore (1798). By 1875, all existing states had health departments.
     c. Early health departments focused on environmental hazards resulting from overcrowding and poor living conditions.
  3. A chronology of nursing leaders and important scientists, since the 1800s (Display 2-1)

G. **Modern Aggregate Concerns (1900–Present)**
  1. School health nursing

     a. **One of the first aggregates focused on by public health agencies and nurses**
     b. Largest response occurred in New York City; in one year (1902–1903) reduced the number of children excluded from school for illnesses from 10,000 to 1000
     c. Began with exclusion and treatment of "nuisance diseases," such as impetigo and ringworm
     d. Incorporated screenings and examinations for treatable conditions such as deficits in growth, vision, and hearing

DISPLAY 2-1.
Leaders in Public Health

1839	Lemuel Shattuck: founded the American Statistical Society and in 1850 called for the government to improve sanitary and social conditions to reduce disease and death.
1842	Edwin Chadwick: wrote a report on the unsanitary conditions among poor persons in England.
1854	John Snow: an English physician; demonstrated that a cholera outbreak was linked to water from the same well.
1856	Florence Nightingale (1820–1910): a trained nurse, the founder of modern nursing; returned from her nursing leadership in the Crimean War and became influential in the development of nursing and nursing education, in addition to her role as nurse researcher and author.
1859	William Rathbone: a wealthy Englishman; was so pleased with the home care of his dying wife, promoted the establishment of a district nursing service. He corresponded regularly with Florence Nightingale and implemented her ideas in the services provided.
1860	Joseph Lister (1827–1912): a British surgeon; developed the technique of antiseptic surgery and washing hands before changing dressings.
1861	Clara Barton (1821–1912): a teacher, not a trained nurse; confronted the unsanitary conditions among Civil War soldiers. One of the founders to the American Red Cross in 1881.
1863	Henri Dunant: founded the International Red Cross, headquartered in Geneva, Switzerland.
1863	Dorothea Dix (1802–1887): a teacher, not a trained nurse; gained prominence for her work in reforming prisons and mental institutions, and was appointed head of the Department of Female Nurses.
1877	Frances Root: the first trained visiting nurse in the United States.
1881	Louis Pasteur (1822–1895): a French chemist and bacteriologist; founded the science of microbiology. He developed the technique of immunization (1881) and produced vaccines (rabies–1885)—both major public health accomplishments.
1882	Robert Koch (1843–1910): a German bacteriologist; applied Pasteur's theories and developed methods for handling and studying bacteria. He discovered cholera and the tubercle bacillus, yet his ideas about TB prevention were not readily instituted.
1893	Lillian Wald (1867–1940): founder of the Henry Street Settlement and the Visiting Nurse Service of New York City, first coined the term *public health nurse*.
1893	Mary Brewster: a nursing student colleague of Lillian Wald; worked with her in developing the Henry Street Settlement.
1893	Isabel Hampton Robb: established the nursing organization that later became the National League for Nursing.
1895	Ada Stewart: a trained visiting nurse; hired by the Vermont Marble Works, to care for sick employees and their families. Considered the first industrial nurse in the United States.
1902	Linda Rogers: a public health nurse working with Lillian Wald; became part of a school nursing experiment in the New York City Health Department and the first school nurse.
1920	C. E. A. Winslow (1877–1957): a leading theoretician of the American public health movement; provided a definition of public health.
1925	Mary Breckenridge (1881–1965): devoted her life to establishing the Frontier Nursing Service, visiting rural Kentucky residents on horseback.

e. Worked with and taught teachers and parent associations about group health

f. Initially focused on elementary schools, and later included high schools

2. Occupational health nursing

a. 1895: industrial nursing grew slowly to other industries in the country as a result of the first industrial nursing success.

b. World War I: increase in hired industrial nurses to meet the demands of industrial growth and manufacturing. By 1919, there were 1200 nurses working in 871 industries.

c. Services focused on first aid, group health teaching on safety and sanitation, visiting sick employees at home, and initiating other services needed (making referrals).

3. Infant–child health nursing

a. 1800s: efforts to improve the health of infants and children (breastfeeding was encouraged, pasteurization of milk provided a clean milk supply to children, and infant day nurseries started)

b. The early 1900s: saw the addition of school nurses, infant clinics, and additional visiting nurses hired solely for infant welfare work

c. **1912: government created the Children's Bureau designed to reduce childhood morbidity and mortality by promoting prenatal care, vaccination, immunization, provision of sanitary milk, and prompt medical care**

4. Tuberculosis (TB) nursing

a. **Primary cause of death among young and middle-age adults at the turn of the 20th century**

b. Also known as *consumption* (because the people seemed to be consumed by the disease as they lost large amounts of weight)

c. Prevention of TB: taught by newly hired nurses in the early 1900s; became a major service provided by visiting nurses associations (VNAs), and remains so today

d. The nurse's role: included prevention, skin testing, and physical care of the ill TB patient

5. Rural nursing

a. Advocated by Lillian Wald

b. The Red Cross Rural Nursing Service: a forerunner of the Public Health Service's work on Indian reservations

c. The Metropolitan Life Insurance Company Visiting Nursing Service: visiting nurses sent to the homes of poor, working class policy holders to improve their health

d. **The Frontier Nursing Service: delivered care to women and children in the underserved, rural areas of eastern Kentucky**

Bibliography

Polgar, S. (1964). Evolution and the ills of mankind. In Tax, S. (Ed.) *Horizons of anthropology,* pp. 200–211. Chicago: Aldine.

Rosen, G. (1958). *A history of public health.* New York: MD Publications, Inc.

Smith, C. M., & Maurer, F. A. (1995). *Community health nursing: Theory and practice.* Philadelphia: W.B. Saunders.

Spradley, B. W., & Allender, J. A. (1996). *Community health nursing: Concepts and practice.* (4th ed.). Philadelphia: Lippincott-Raven.

Swanson, J. M., & Albrecht, M. (1993). *Community health nursing: Promoting the health of aggregates.* Philadelphia: W.B. Saunders.

Thomas, C. L. (Ed.) (1993) *Taber's cyclopedic medical dictionary* (17th ed.). Philadelphia: F.A. Davis.

STUDY QUESTIONS

1. What we know about our forefathers and their health, illness, and accident experiences goes back as far as:
   a. Prehistoric times
   b. 10,000 BC
   c. Biblical times
   d. The 1800s

2. In the industrial era (1600–1900), major health problems included:
   a. Large bowel diseases, such as cancer
   b. Heart disease and vascular problems
   c. Diabetes and other metabolic disorders
   d. Epidemics of communicable diseases

3. Origins of public health efforts can be traced back to:
   a. The Hebrew Hygienic Code
   b. Primitive societies
   c. Egypt and the Middle East
   d. Greece and Rome

4. During the Middle Ages (500–1500 AD), communicable diseases grew to epidemic proportions. A major cause of this was:
   a. The Crusades
   b. Monasteries
   c. Leprosy
   d. Religious influences

5. During the 1800s, many achievements occurred to promote public health. The crowning achievement of that time was the:
   a. Discovery of the microscope
   b. Discovery of the germ theory
   c. Building of the first hospitals
   d. Elimination of immigration

6. Which nurse coined the term *public health nurse*, established the Henry Street Settlement, and is also known as the founder of public health nursing?
   a. Clara Barton
   b. Dorothea Dix
   c. Mary Breckenridge
   d. Lillian Wald

7. The advent of school nursing occurred when:
   a. Organized schooling began in the United States
   b. Absenteeism was high among immigrant children in New York City
   c. Occupational health nursing spilled over into the schools
   d. A large number of birth defects were noticed in school-age children

8. Nursing services to the employed in the United States first began by Ada Stewart at the:
   a. Triangle Shirt Company
   b. Metropolitan Insurance Company
   c. Vermont Marble Company
   d. Lippincott-Raven Publishing Company

9. A special aggregate to receive public health nursing services in 1900 were those with TB. This came about because tuberculosis was:
   a. The primary cause of death among adults in 1900
   b. Killing newborns faster than any other cause
   c. A new disease just beginning to affect people in the United States
   d. Causing high absenteeism in elementary school children

10. The Frontier Nursing Service brought nursing services to people living in rural:
    a. Indian reservations
    b. Eastern Kentucky
    c. Colorado mountains
    d. Plains states

ANSWER KEY

1. **Correct response: a**
   The other choices depict more recent years. Our knowledge of people on this earth goes back to prehistoric humans.
   Comprehension/NA/NA

2. **Correct response: d**
   During the industrial era, major epidemics took many lives. Answer choices **a, b,** and **c** represent the health problems of the modern era (after 1900) when we began to conquer communicable diseases of the day.
   Comprehension/NA/NA

3. **Correct response: b**
   The earliest public health efforts are documented among people in primitive societies. The responses in answer choices **a, c,** and **d** occurred later. Each era contributed practices that have improved public health efforts.
   Comprehension/NA/NA

4. **Correct response: a**
   During the Crusades, thousands of people traveled across Europe and the Middle East to enlighten people in the name of religion. However, through these travels they brought many new communicable diseases to people never exposed before.
   b. Monasteries offered a refuge for the sick.
   c. Leprosy had been around for thousands of years before this time and was just one of many illnesses affecting the population.
   d. Although religion influenced how people were treated, religion did not cause illnesses.
   Comprehension/NA/NA

5. **Correct response: b**
   The discovery and acceptance of the germ theory changed the approach of public health measures and opened the door to future discoveries that would

lead to the eradication of many diseases.
   a. The microscope was invented centuries earlier. It was enhanced and begun to be used by scientists in the 1800s.
   c. The early hospitals were monasteries. Building of asylums and hospitals began in the 1600s and 1700s.
   d. Actually immigration was at a peak in the 1800s, especially the last 25 years of that century.
   Comprehension/NA/NA

6. **Correct response: d**
   a. Clara Barton was a teacher and volunteer nurse, and is known for being the founder of the American Red Cross.
   b. Dorothea Dix was a teacher who committed her life to prison and mental health reform.
   c. Mary Breckenridge was a nurse-midwife who founded the Frontier Nursing Service in Kentucky.
   Comprehension/NA/NA

7. **Correct response: b**
   a. Schools existed in the United States since the 1600s. School nursing began at the turn of the 20th century in 1902.
   c. Occupational health nursing (industrial nursing) and school nursing began about the same time and one did not necessarily influence the other.
   d. There were no significant increases in birth defects noted. What was noted was communicable diseases and other ills of poverty and overcrowding.
   Comprehension/Health Promotion/ Assessment

8. *Correct response: c*
   a. This company had a disastrous fire, which killed many young female workers early in the 1900s. They had no industrial nursing services.
   b. This insurance company started a home nursing service to its policy-holders early in the 1900s, but not occupational nursing services.
   d. This publishing company has been in existence since the 1700s but did not have the first occupational nursing services.

Comprehension/NA/NA

9. *Correct response: a*
   b. TB was not a major killer of infants at the turn of the century.

   c. TB was a classic communicable disease, occurring more frequently as people began living closer together.
   d. Absenteeism from school occurred from "nuisance" diseases such as lice, scabies, impetigo, and so forth. TB did not affect the young child as much as it affected young adults.

Comprehension/NA/NA

10. *Correct response: b*
    a, c, and **d** are locations needing public health services but were not among the service areas of the Frontier Nursing Service.

Comprehension/NA/NA

An Overview of Community Health Care Systems

3

I. A Global View of Community Health Care Systems
A. World Health Organization (WHO)

1. Created as an agency of the United Nations, a coalition of 61 national governments formed in 1945. Membership increased to 168 members by 1988.

2. WHO's *goal* is to attain the highest possible level of health for all, and its *mission* is to be the one directing and coordinating authority on international health.

3. WHO is headquartered in Geneva, Switzerland and provides eight basic health care services to member nations (Display 3-1).

DISPLAY 3-1.
The Eight Basic Health Care Services Identified
by the World Health Organization (WHO, 1978)

> ► Education about prevailing health problems, including methods of prevention and control
> ► Promotion of adequate food supply and proper nutrition
> ► Provision of safe water and basic sanitation
> ► Administration of maternal and child health care, including family planning
> ► Immunization against the major infectious diseases
> ► Prevention and control of locally endemic diseases
> ► Appropriate treatment of common diseases and injuries
> ► Provision of essential drugs

4.   WHO provides technical services, information from epidemiology and statistics, advising and consulting, and demonstration teams.

B.   Pan-American Health Organization (PAHO)

1.   The oldest continuously functioning international health organization in the world, PAHO was founded in 1902.

2.   PAHO became one of the six regional offices of WHO and is located in Washington, DC.

3.   PAHO is the central coordinating organization for public health in the Western Hemisphere.

C.   Other International Organizations

1.   International Red Cross is a major voluntary agency that provides services to people during war and disasters and to those in military service.

   a.   The American Red Cross, a branch of the International Red Cross, established in 1882 by Clara Barton is a quasi-official agency (mandated by the US government to provide certain services, but receives no federal funds)

   b.   Provides disaster relief and other health (blood supply), education (safety and first aid), and counseling services

2.   UNICEF

   a.   Initially established as an emergency relief program for children in war-torn areas

   b.   Currently promotes child and maternal health in the world through a variety of programs and activities

3.   Additional programs

   a.   Government programs: ACTION (houses the Peace Corps), Office of International Health in the Department of Health and Human Services

   b.   Private agencies: Project HOPE and the International Planned Parenthood Federation

II. The National View of Community Health Systems in the United States

    A. Legislation Enacting Health Care Services (1921–1946)

        1. Shepard-Towner Act of 1921 provided federal funds to the states for programs to promote the health of mothers and infants

            a. Targeted prematurity, perinatal mortality, nutrition, mental retardation, audiology, rheumatic fever, cerebral palsy, epilepsy, dentistry, delinquency, and migrant child health

            b. Set a pattern for maternal and child health programs

        2. Social Security Act of 1935 had a tremendous impact on public health

            a. **Provides welfare insurance and assistance that benefits high-risk mothers and children, disabled, and aged**

            b. **Strengthened local health departments and programs**

        3. Hill-Burton Act of 1946 was the first national health facilities planning act linking health planning with comprehensive population needs, providing federal funds to states for hospital construction

    B. Legislation Enacting US Community Health Systems (1965–1987)

        1. Sedicare-Medicaid—1965 (Table 3-1)

            a. **Medicare—Title XVIII of the Social Security Act—provides federally funded health insurance for elderly (65 and over) and the disabled, regardless of their income level.**

            b. **Medicaid—Title XIX of the Social Security Act—a joint federal–state health insurance program serving the aged, blind, disabled, and families with dependent children who meet low-income parameters**

        2. The Occupational Safety and Health Act (OSHA) enacted in 1970 provides protection to private industry and federal government workers against personal injury or illness occurring from hazardous working conditions

            a. County or municipal employees are covered by state safety and health organizations

            b. In work settings with few employees, the workers are not protected by health and safety regulations

        3. The Omnibus Budget Reconciliation Act (OBRA) of 1981 was enacted as a federal budget control measure

            a. OBRA severely affected funding of public health services that had been enacted in the previous 45 years

            b. Amendments were added to OBRA in 1987 to increase quality control in nursing homes and home care

TABLE 3-1.
Medicare/Medicaid Comparison

MEDICARE*	MEDICAID*
TITLE XVIII OF THE SOCIAL SECURITY ACT	TITLE XIX OF THE SOCIAL SECURITY ACT
1. Medicare is a national health insurance program for people 65 years of age and older, certain younger disabled people, and people with kidney failure.	1. Medicaid receives federal and state money to provide health care to people living below a certain income level.
2. It is divided into two parts. Hospital Insurance (Part A) helps pay for hospital care, skilled nursing facilities, home health, and hospice care. Medical Insurance (Part B) helps pay doctor bills, outpatient hospital care and various other medical services not covered by Part A.	2. The program is managed differently in each state; benefits may fluctuate as well as differ state to state. Services covered are based on state health care priorities and needs of those most eligible, such as pregnant women, infants, children, the disabled, and the elderly.
3. Eligibility includes age, 10 years of Medicare-covered employment, citizenship or permanent resident status.	3. People over age 65 who meet income and asset guidelines are eligible for Medicare and Medicaid.
4. Part A is free whereas Part B had a monthly premium in 1997 of $43.80. (This is deducted from the Social Security, Railroad Retirement, or Civil Service Retirement check.)	4. Some people in higher low-income brackets have a copayment, which means they pay a certain amount of the cost of the health care service they receive or they may have to spend so much on health care costs in a month before Medicaid begins to pay.
5. Medicare does not cover all the health care costs. It is estimated that Medicare alone only covers about 40% of the costs of health-related services elders experience.	5. Medicaid covers health care costs similar to Medicare. However, because they are different in each state and may change month by month it is important for the recipient or health care provider to verify coverage with the office managing the program.
6. Elders are advised to buy supplemental insurance called a "Medigap" policy. There are several plans from which to choose.	
7. The Social Security Administration can answer questions about Medicare. Toll free phone number: 1-800-772-1213. (7AM–7PM)	

*Both Medicare and Medicaid are moving into the managed care arena, which affects accessibility and services for clients.

4. Public Law 98-12—Diagnostic Related Groups (DRGs) of 1983 amended the Social Security Act and initiated major reforms in health care financing, changing health care payment from retrospective to prospective reimbursement through a classification system of 467 diagnostic related groups.
   a. Medicare and other insurers base reimbursement on a fixed preset rate by diagnosis
   b. DRGs create a positive incentive for hospitals to reduce costs through early hospital discharge

5. The Health Objectives Planning Act of 1990 provided financial support to achieve the goals outlined in the Institute of Medicine's Report Healthy People 2000 (see Chap. 18). In 1991, funding was increased for health promotion and disease prevention to assist in meeting the goals

C. Federal Health Agencies

1. The Department of Health and Human Services (DHHS) is the agency most involved with the health and welfare of US citizens (Display 3-2).

2. DHHS services at the federal level that directly impact the role of the community health nurse (CHN) include:

   a. Conducting research and research-related training through the National Center for Nursing Research, within the National Institutes of Health
   b. Providing statistics and consultation services
   c. Providing technical assistance to public and private organizations
   d. Providing professional nursing expertise and leadership
   e. Assisting in planning ways to improve nursing services
   f. Fostering, supporting, and conducting projects to expand nursing's scientific base

 3. DHHS services provide planning, consultation, and support to the state level of services but no direct care to clients

D. State Health Services

1. State health departments—typically state health department services are focused on planning, consulting, and supporting local agencies and providing indirect care to clients. Services include:

   a. Maintaining intergovernmental and other agency relations

DISPLAY 3-2.
The Department of Health and Human Services

1. Office of Human Development Services
2. Social Security Administration
3. Health Care Financing and Administration
4. Public Health Service
   ► Health Resources and Services Administration, Bureau of Health Professions, Division of Nursing
   ► Agency for Health Care Policy and Research
   ► Agency for Toxic Substances and Disease Registry
   ► Alcohol, Drug Abuse, and Mental Health Administration
   ► Centers for Disease Control and Prevention
   ► Food and Drug Administration
   ► Indian Health Service
   ► National Institutes of Health

              b.   Regulating health services

              c.   Compiling vital records and statistics

              d.   Providing statewide health planning and development

              e.   Setting standards

        2.   State Education Departments

              a.   Responsible for coordinating health curricula and services provided within local school systems

              b.   Using CHNs on councils to facilitate joint coordination within and between school districts, and to develop policy and guidelines for school health services and health education

        3.   State Department of Corrections

              a.   CHNs work as planners and coordinators of service

              b.   CHNs supervise health and nursing services for inmates in some state prisons; in others, the state contracts for health care from private companies who provide nurses for prison employment

  E. **Local Health Care Services**

        1.   Typical county and city health department services include:

              a.   Health planning and administration

              b.   Environmental health services

              c.   Prevention and control of communicable diseases

              d.   Public health nursing services

              e.   Personal health services

        2.   **At the local level, clients receive direct services**

III. **Issues Affecting US Community Health Care Systems**

  A. **Aging and Longevity**

        1.   The fastest growing group of people are those over 65

        2.   Immunizations, antibiotics, preventive health care practices of incorporating good nutrition and exercise, and organ transplants have added years to people's lives

  B. **Chronic Illnesses**

        1.   Heart disease, cancer, diabetes, hypertension, and COPD are common diseases elders manage and live with

        2.   Years of managing the cost of these diseases strain personal, state, and national budgets

        3.   As people live longer, this will continue to be a major health care issue that CHNs will manage

  C. **Quality and Cost of Health Care**

        1.   Managed care solution: A system that coordinates medical care for specific groups to promote provider efficiency and control costs. This eliminates duplication of services and aims to prevent gaps in health care. However, in containing costs, some managed care systems may be decreasing the quality of care they provide.

2. Clinical pathways: A system of identified objectives to guide caregiving, with distinct time limits, that focuses on quality care, measurable goals, and client outcomes.

3. Community partnerships: Establishing relationships in the community with businesses, universities, schools, health departments, hospitals, and industries to maximize client care and minimize costs.

D. Immigration—Shifting Populations and Their Needs

1. In some communities, increasing numbers of immigrants (legal and illegal) and refugees impact health and health care services:
   a. Economics—increased demand for services exceeds funds and staff available
   b. Cultural—challenges providers to deliver appropriate care, which includes translators, dietary modifications, and resources as needed
   c. Illegal immigration—because illegal immigrants bypass health requirements, they may be in fragile health states and a source of communicable diseases

2. In states most affected by illegal immigration, the cost of providing health and related educational and welfare services imposes economic and political challenges that can divide the community

E. Societal Problems

1. Types of societal problems
   a. Violence
   b. Crime
   c. Gangs
   d. Poverty
   e. Homelessness
   f. Teenage pregnancy
   g. Divorce/single parenting
   h. Ineffective parenting skills
   i. Gay and lesbian rights
   j. Substance abuse
   k. High-risk lifestyle issues

2. Effects on health care
   a. *Increased cost*—requiring more money, staff, services, and programs
   b. *Decreased quality of life*—more time spent responding to problems, less time spent on health care services that focus on primary preventive activities that are more productive for society

      c. *Expanded demand for services*—increases and overburdens local agencies, which, again, increases costs

IV. The Community Health Nurse as a Political Influence

  A. **Writing to Legislators**

      1. Purpose: sway public officials' view toward or against a particular position

      2. Implementation: express personal opinion and provide useful data (legislators often read personal communication); avoid form letters (they are tallied by an administrative assistant)

  B. **Visiting Legislators**

      1. Purpose: make a personal appeal for or against a particular issue coming before the legislator in order to sway his/her vote

      2. Implementation: send a briefing sheet or letter before the visit. Time will be limited. If you can only get to see a staff member, this may still be worthwhile. They may know more of the details about a bill and may have more time than the legislator.

  C. **Attending Hearings or Testifying**

      1. Purpose: impact decisions on a pending bill or proposed legislation

      2. Implementation: alone or as a group, the nurse's presence communicates concern and a readiness for action. Testimony can be provided verbally or in writing

  D. **Involving Interdisciplinary Teams in Health Promotion**

      1. Team composition: legislators, council members, mayors and other people in politically powerful positions listen to doctors, nurses, educators, social workers, and others who are knowledgeable about the health and welfare issues. An interdisciplinary team can exert a powerful influence. (See example in Display 3-3.)

      2. Purpose: involving interdisciplinary health team members who interact with political leaders gives the broader community view

---

DISPLAY 3-3.
An Interdisciplinary Team Can Make a Difference

Example—A bill is coming before the state legislature prohibiting high school students with epilepsy from enrolling in driver's education classes if they have had seizures after age 12. With this new bill, even if a teen has been seizure free for 3 years, he or she must wait until age 18 to take driver's education. The professional advisory board from the local chapter of the Epilepsy Foundation met with the district's state legislator to convince him of the drawbacks of this new bill. The advisory council has members from different disciplines—a pharmacist, a community health nurse, a school nurse, a pharmaceutical salesperson, a neurologist, and the agency's executive director. This group of people presented a powerful argument with statistics, current literature, and personal testimony from each point of view, which gave the legislator the background needed to intelligently support defeat of the bill. Several of the members were invited to give testimony at a hearing on this issue. The bill did not pass.

of an issue, which enables the legislator to consider the issue from a variety of views

3. Implementation: interdisciplinary health team meets to plan strategy, contacts various community political leaders' offices and, in groups of various sizes, meet with the leaders to present their collective views

E. Empowering Community Members

1. Purpose: enable groups in the community to express concerns effectively and to bring about community changes that promote their well-being

 2. Implementation:

  a. **Educate key community leaders in the political process**
  b. **Assist the community members to define their own needs**
  c. **Be available as a consultant; allow leadership to come from within the group**
  d. **Know when to step back and give ownership to the group. Success occurs when the nurse is no longer needed—this is the nurse's goal**

Bibliography

Spradley, B. W., & Allender, J. A. (1996). *Community health nursing: Concepts and practice.* (4th ed.). Philadelphia: Lippincott-Raven.

Stanhope, M., & Lancaster, J. (1992). *Community health nursing: Process and practice for promoting health.* (3rd ed.). St. Louis: Mosby–Year Book.

World Health Organization. (1978). *Primary health care.* Geneva: WHO.

Your Medicare Handbook, 1996. (1996, April). Pub. No. HCFA-10050. Baltimore, MD: Health Care Financing Administration.

STUDY QUESTIONS

1. The mission of the World Health Organization (WHO) states it aims to:
   a. Have all countries in the world become member nations
   b. Be the one authority on international health
   c. Eradicate smallpox from the globe
   d. Set up free-standing clinics in all communities of member nations

2. The Pan-American Health Organization is:
   a. A new agency organized to provide care in Central America
   b. The "umbrella organization" directing world health services
   c. The oldest of the six regional offices of the WHO
   d. An organization in competition with the WHO

3. The *first* act to provide federal funds to the states for programs to promote the health of mothers and infants was the:
   a. Shepard-Towner Act
   b. Social Security Act
   c. Hill-Burton Act
   d. Occupational Safety and Health Act

4. Title XVIII of the Social Security Act provided funding for health insurance for the elderly and permanently disabled. This program is called:
   a. Medicaid
   b. Medicare
   c. Diagnostic Related Groups
   d. Social Security

5. Title XIX of the Social Security Act provides funding for health care to people in low-income categories, regardless of age. This program is called:
   a. Medicaid
   b. Medicare
   c. Diagnostic Related Groups
   d. Social Security

6. At the federal level, community health care is administered through the following operating component of the Department of Health and Human Services:
   a. Social Security Administration
   b. Health Care Financing and Administration
   c. Office of Human Development Services
   d. Public Health Services

7. At the local level of health care, the services that can be expected fall in the category of:
   a. Indirect—such as consultation and support
   b. Direct—such as clinic and individual health care services
   c. Funding—provides the money and resources for services
   d. Planning—for the services needed in the nation

8. Major issues affecting the US community health care system include:
   a. An aging society, with multiple chronic illnesses
   b. A shortening life span among men and women
   c. Stabilization of immigration into the United States
   d. A nationwide decrease in crime and violence

9. When writing letters to legislators, you should remember to:
   a. Use form letters for consistency and easy tabulation
   b. Not express personal opinion. It is viewed negatively by legislators
   c. Speak positively on an issue, not negatively
   d. Express personal opinion and provide useful data

10. Empowering community members includes the following activities on the part of the CHN:
    a. Doing all of the activities for the community members
    b. Stepping back at the beginning and giving little input
    c. Giving the ownership and leadership to the community
    d. Defining the community needs for the members

ANSWER KEY

1. *Correct response: b*
  a. This is not spelled out in their mission and would be a monumental task.
  c. Smallpox has been eradicated from the earth since the 1980s.
  d. The WHO works with member nations to provide individualized forms of health care delivery, based on each nation's needs.
Comprehension/Health Promotion/ Assessment

2. *Correct response: c*
  a. The PAHO is the oldest (1902) regional office of the WHO and provides health care services to all of the Americas and Canada, not just Central America.
  b. The WHO is the "umbrella" organization for the six regional offices; PAHO is one regional office.
  d. The PAHO is a part of WHO, not a competing organization.
Comprehension/NA/NA

3. *Correct response: a. This act was the first in 1921 and set a trend to promote the health of mothers and children.*
  b. This 1935 act had broad welfare insurance for many groups, including women and children.
  c. This 1946 act provided federal funds to states for hospital construction.
  d. This 1970 act provided protection from injury and illness while at work.
Comprehension/NA/NA

4. *Correct response: b*
  a. This is Title XIX of the Social Security Act and provides health care to people meeting low-income guidelines, regardless of age.
  c. This is a way of paying for health care, part of a prospective payment system.
  d. This is the basic act that Title XVIII is a part of.
Comprehension/NA/NA

5. *Correct response: a*
  b. This is Title XVIII of the Social Security Act and provides health insurance to the elderly and the permanently disabled.
  c. This is a way of paying for health care, part of a prospective payment system.
  d. This is the basic act that Title XIX is a part of.
Comprehension/NA/NA

6. *Correct response: d*
  a, b, and **c** are the other three operating components of the DHHS. Community health care concerns are administrated through the Public Health Service.
Comprehension/NA/NA

7. *Correct response: b*
  a. This describes the services offered by the state level of government.
  c. This describes one of the main services offered by the federal level of government.
  d. Planning is another important service of the federal level of government.
Comprehension/NA/Assessment

8. *Correct response: a*
  b. The life span of men and women is slowly increasing; it is not decreasing.
  c. Immigration into the United States continues to increase. Regulation for legal immigration has been in effect for decades, however, some states experience uncontrolled illegal immigration.
  d. Unfortunately, crime and violence continue to be community health problems and are in epidemic proportions in some communities.
Comprehension/NA/Analysis

9. *Correct response: d*
    a. Form letters are not recommended. Legislators tend not to read them.
    b. Personal opinion is desired and the purpose of writing.
    c. Negative and positive comments are welcomed and needed to sway a vote.

Comprehension/NA/Analysis

10. *Correct response: c*
    a. The CHN should encourage the community members to become involved, and most of the needed activities are carried out by them.
    b. Stepping back prematurely may not achieve the goals of an empowered community. Stepping back comes later in the process.
    d. The community defines its own needs.

Comprehension/Safe Care/Planning

Unit II
The Community as Client

Community Assessments: A Basis for Community Health Nursing

I. Definitions of a Community

A. *A Physically Focused Definition:* "A locality-based entity, composed of interdependent systems of formal organizations reflecting societal institutions, informal groups, and aggregates, and whose function or expressed intent is to meet a wide variety of collective needs. The target of community-oriented practice." (Stanhope & Lancaster, 1992)

B. *A People-Focused Definition:* "A community is a collection of people who interact with each other and whose common interests or characteristics give them a sense of unity and belonging." (Spradley & Allender, 1996)

C.   *A Comprehensive Definition:* "An open social system characterized by people in a place over time who have common goals." (Smith & Maurer, 1995)

D.   *Definition of a Healthy Community:* "Healthy communities are able to collaborate effectively in identifying the problems and needs of the community, can achieve a working consensus on goals and priorities, can agree on ways and means to implement the agreed-on goals, and can collaborate effectively in the required actions." (Cottrell, 1976)

 II.   The Three Dimensions of a Community

A.   *A Location:* or geographic location where this community exists such as *California State University, Fresno, California.* With this community's location, you get the state, city, and university. The health of this community is affected by its location, and the community health nurse (CHN) needs to know that location includes:

1.   Boundary of the community
2.   Placement of health services
3.   Geographic features
4.   Climate
5.   Plants and animals
6.   Human-made environment

B.   *A Population:* encompasses the population of the entire community including all the diverse people within the boundaries of the community. In the above example, this includes the students, staff, faculty, and visitors. It is important for the CHN to be aware of population variables, such as:

1.   Size
2.   Density
3.   Composition
4.   Rate of growth or decline
5.   Cultural characteristics
6.   Social class
7.   Mobility

C.   *A Social System:* every community has a social system with various parts that interact and influence the larger system. In the example, a university has: admissions, food service, health services, the library, classrooms of different sizes and types, dormitories, financial aid, administration, and so forth. The variables include the following systems:

1.   Health
2.   Family
3.   Economic

      4. Educational
      5. Religious
      6. Welfare
      7. Political
      8. Recreational
      9. Legal
    10. Communication

III. Purposes of Community Assessments

A. To determine the strengths, weaknesses, and needs of communities

B. To establish a knowledge base of community resources

C. To determine the needs and resources of specific subpopulations

IV. Methods of Community Assessments (Display 4-1)

A. Familiarization (Overview or "Windshield Survey")

    1. Helps the CHN become familiar with the data available in the community

    2. Enables the CHN to gain a working knowledge of the community

    3. Is necessary for the CHN to work effectively with families, groups, organizations, and populations

    4. Requires that CHNs drive around the community and locate major business, religious, social, government, and health resources and introduce themselves to key community members as a new CHN working in the area

B. Comprehensive

    1. Is the most thorough of all the assessment types

    2. Is the most traditional, most time consuming, and most expensive

    3. The total community is assessed in terms of geographic, population, political-social, and resources or liabilities. The impact of the surrounding area on the community of interest is considered.

    4. Is conducted to identify potential health problems and to validate actual problems

    5. Is conducted using:

       a. Available data (gathered from interviews, community forums, statistics collected by official agencies, such as census data)

       b. Interviews of key informants

       c. Surveys compiled by the CHN

    6. Has inherent problems and is seldom done because of the expense and resource-intensive nature of the comprehensive assessment, a more focused approach, such as the problem-oriented, or subsystem assessment is preferred by staff CHNs

DISPLAY 4-1.
Examples of Community Assessments

Familiarization: A nurse is hired by a local health department. He is new to the community. During his first week of orientation, he spends 1 day driving around the community, introducing himself to the staff in the schools, managers of businesses, and the clergy. He gathers literature about special services, gets phone numbers, and leaves his business card. He begins to feel like a part of his new community.

Problem-oriented: One of the nurses in the health department has just visited a family new to the community. A 6-year-old child has a distinct speech problem. The nurse is not familiar with all the re-sources in the community for speech development. She conducts a problem-oriented assessment. She be-gins by exploring services she is aware of at the local hospital and talking with the school nurse. This leads her to programs at a neighboring college, available financial assistance through special childrens' services, several dentists specializing in orthodontics, and the school speech pathologist. From these con-tacts, she has developed a list of regional and national resources she intends to contact. Now she has the information she needs to assist this family.

Comprehensive Assessment: The Valley Indian Health Program has an opportunity to receive a major federal grant ($100,000 for 5 years) to assist high-risk families of Native American origin. The five community health nurses in the agency begin to write the grant but need comprehensive information about their community to accompany the grant application. To gather these data they rely on available data from the Federal Bureau of Indian Affairs and local census data, they interview tribal leaders, and they develop a survey to give to as many young families as they can at clinic visits and on home visits the nurses make. They also distributed the surveys at a Pow-Wow, a major Native American social event. Working together, they were able to meet the deadline with the assessment data required for this grant.

Subsystem Assessment: The nurses at Valley Indian Health are so busy no one nurse could devote the time needed to complete the comprehensive assessment. However, as a group of five, they divided the community into subsystems such as tribal elders, teenagers, newborns (high-risk populations); clinical services available (dental, prenatal, etc.), community resources (specific financial and material resources available for subsystem populations), each taking one or two, and they were able to focus their data gath-ering on the specific subsystems. This achieved their goal, yet did not overburden any one nurse. They met on several occasions to share the data as they worked on writing the grant. Because they are in competi-tion for the money, they may not receive the grant. Nevertheless, they now have a more thorough knowl-edge of their community from the comprehensiveness of doing several subsystem assessments.

7.   May be conducted by advanced practice nurses, interprofes-sional teams, and with grant support

C.   **Problem-Oriented**

1.   **Focuses on a specific topic, a particular health problem or social issue that relates to the health of a group**

2.   **Assesses the community in relation to the identified problem**

3.   **Is more limited than the others, with energies focused on one issue, thus making it more cost-effective than a com-prehensive assessment, and is used for a different purpose than the familiarization assessment**

4.   **Assists the nurse by providing data necessary for plan-ning to address the selected problem**

D. Subsystem
1. Focuses on a single aspect of the community such as its formal political, school, religious system, or population groups
2. Can be conducted by a team of people, each assessing one or two subsystems. The combined information would give more thorough community assessment data

V. Assessment Methods
A. Surveys
1. Written or verbal
2. The CHN investigator can use existing or newly developed surveys.
3. Surveys can be completed by telephone or in person on home or clinic visits, at immunization programs, or in public settings, such as at shopping malls or county fairs.

B. Interviews
1. Usually more comprehensive than a survey
2. They are done verbally, in person, and are designed to obtain detailed information from a key person's perspective.
3. The key person may be a community leader or the potential recipient of services. Each will give a different perspective on the same issue. All views are needed to get a total view of the problem.

C. Community Forum
1. This is an ideal way to get community input because it is cost-effective and has broad participation.
2. A convenient location is secured, many community members are invited, and the forum is conducted by someone with knowledge of the issues and an ability and interest to address large groups.
3. Community members share opinions about needs, services, or specific topics they want to address. The leader may focus the topic discussion to get more depth or the broader community perspective.
4. Another type of forum is the focus group. This is a smaller group (7 to 10 members), and the group is charged with intense discussion on all aspects of one particular issue. Holding more than one focus group helps to identify patterns in perception.

VI. Sources for Community Assessment Data: These data sources can be obtained at the library.
A. National Center for Health Statistics, Hyattsville, MD
1. Vital Statistics of the United States
2. Monthly Vital Statistics Report
3. Vital and Health Statistics Service

B. **Bureau of the Census, Washington, DC**
   1. Current Population Reports, Series P-25
   2. Current Population Reports, Series P-23, Special Studies

 C. **Public Health Service, Centers for Disease Control and Prevention—Morbidity and Mortality Weekly Report (MMWR)**

VII. The Characteristics of a Healthy Community (Cottrell, 1976)
   A. Effective collaboration in identifying community needs and problems
   B. Achievement of a working consensus on goals and priorities
   C. Agreement on ways and means to implement the agreed-upon goals
   D. Effective collaboration in the required actions

 VIII. Descriptors of a Healthy Community
   A. One in which members have a high degree of awareness that "we are a community"
   B. Uses its natural resources while taking steps to conserve them for future generations
   C. Openly recognizes the existence of subgroups and welcomes their participation in community affairs
   D. Prepared to meet crises
   E. A problem-solving community; it identifies, analyzes, and organizes to meet its own needs
   F. Has open channels of communication that allow information to flow among all subgroups of citizens in all directions
   G. Seeks to make each of its systems' resources available to all members of the community
   H. Has legitimate and effective ways to settle disputes that arise within the community
   I. Encourages maximum citizen participation in decision making
   J. Promotes a high level of wellness among all its members (Spradley & Allender, 1996)

Bibliography

Cottrell, L. S., Jr. (1976). The competent community. In B. H. Kaplan, R. N. Wilson, & A. H. Leighton (Eds.). *Further explorations in social psychiatry* (pp. 195–209). New York: Basic Books.

Smith, C. M., & Maurer, F. A. (1995). *Community health nursing: Theory and practice.* Philadelphia: W.B. Saunders.

Spradley, B. W., & Allender, J. A. (1996). *Community health nursing: Concepts and practice.* (4th ed.). Philadelphia: Lippincott-Raven

Stanhope, M., & Lancaster, J. (1992). *Community health nursing: Process and practice for promoting health.* (3rd ed.). St. Louis: Mosby–Year Book.

Swanson, J. M., & Albrecht, M. (1993). *Community health nursing: Promoting the health of aggregates.* Philadelphia: W.B. Saunders.

STUDY QUESTIONS

1. A physically focused definition of a community suggests that it is composed of:
   a. Interdependent societal institutions, informal groups and aggregates
   b. A collection of people who interact with each other
   c. People working together on the required actions to reach goals and priorities
   d. Interests and characteristics that give it a sense of unity and belonging

2. There are dimensions common to communities, which include:
   a. Money, buildings, and power
   b. Status, equipment, and resources
   c. Location, population, and a social system
   d. Water, land, and a source of energy

3. The purpose of conducting a community assessment includes:
   a. Satisfying one's curiosity about a particular place
   b. Looking for one particular client family you will be visiting
   c. Making travel in the community easier in the future
   d. Determining strengths, weaknesses, needs, and resources

4. A community assessment where the nurse drives around the community and explores resources and introduces himself or herself to key community leaders is called a:
   a. Familiarization, orientation, or "windshield survey" assessment
   b. Comprehensive assessment
   c. Problem-oriented assessment
   d. Subsystem assessment

5. The nurse is exploring the teen pregnancy issue in her community. She does a community assessment that focuses on all factors in this community contributing to this issue. This is a:
   a. Familiarization, orientation, or "windshield survey" assessment

   b. Comprehensive assessment
   c. Problem-oriented assessment
   d. Subsystem assessment

6. The CHN explores each of the three dimensions of the community and uses data in existence, in addition to information gathered from community leaders and community members. The nurse explores all subsystems. This is a:
   a. Familiarization, orientation or "windshield" assessment
   b. Comprehensive assessment
   c. Problem-oriented assessment
   d. Subsystem assessment

7. A method of gathering data for a community assessment that includes a written questionnaire given to clients attending the well child clinic at the health department is an example of a(n):
   a. Survey
   b. Interview
   c. Community forum
   d. Focus group

8. A nurse secures the auditorium of the local high school and invites the elders to attend a meeting in the early evening. The topic to be discussed is the health care needs of older adults as perceived by those in attendance and whether they are being met or not in the services provided by the community. This is an example of a(n):
   a. Survey
   b. Interview
   c. Community forum
   d. Focus group

9. The CHN asks for the elders to meet with her in smaller meetings of 7 to 10 members. At these smaller meetings, she selects some of the key issues discussed in the larger group and asks for their thoughts on the subject. She holds several of these meetings with different elders. From this information, she gets the perceptions of a cross section of elders. This is an example of a(n):

a. Survey
b. Interview
c. Community forum
d. Focus group

10. Descriptors of a healthy community include:
    a. A community where the members are disease free

b. Seeking to make its resources available to all members
c. The leaders making the decisions for community members
d. Keeping subgroups informed of community changes when necessary

ANSWER KEY

1. *Correct response: a*
   b. This response is from the people-focused definition by Spradley & Allender, 1996.
   c. **and** d. are responses from the definition of a healthy community from Cottrell, 1976.
   Comprehension/NA/Analysis

2. *Correct response: c*
   Choices a, b, or d include components of each dimension. For example, in the correct response, a social system is a collective term, so the individual components of power, resources, and a source of energy (each found in one of the other answer choices) may or may not be present in one particular community's social system, but each community *has* a social system.
   Comprehension/NA/Analysis

3. *Correct response: d*
   a. A nurse may be curious about the community but, as he/she assesses the community, the purpose is greater than just curiosity.
   b. This is an expensive way to locate a family and is not done for that purpose.
   c. Perhaps after a community assessment the nurse can travel around a community with greater ease, but the purpose of doing the assessment in the first place was not to make travel easier.
   Application/Health Promotion/ Assessment

4. *Correct response: a.* A new nurse, or a student nurse new to community health nursing, would use this type of assessment to become familiar with the community and be able to start a working relationship with key community leaders.
   Answer choices b, c, and d describe other types of community assessment.
   Application/NA/Assessment

5. *Correct response: c.* The nurse will explore all factors that contribute to the teenage pregnancy issue, and conduct a problem-oriented assessment. The problem is teenage pregnancy. The assessment is problem-oriented.
   Answer choices a, b, and d describe other types of community assessment.
   Application/NA/Assessment

6. *Correct response: b.* The nurse is exploring all subsystems and uses all information available, and new information is gathered. This constitutes a comprehensive assessment, which is very resource-intensive and rarely conducted by staff CHNs.
   Answer choices a, c, and d describe other types of community assessment.
   Application/NA/Assessment

7. *Correct response: a.* This describes a survey, which can be done in writing or verbally, in person or on the telephone. This gives the nurse new data to add to other information as an assessment is being conducted.
   Answer choices b, c, and d describe other methods of data collection.
   Application/NA/Assessment

8. *Correct response: c.* This describes the community forum, where a large group of people are invited to share their views on a subject.
   Answer choices a, b, and d describe other methods of data collection.
   Application/NA/Assessment

9. *Correct response: d.* This example describes the focus group. At focus groups, the nurse gets more detailed information and a cross-section of ideas from the various small groups. This is a valuable tool to begin the planning process of new services.
   Answer choices a, b, and c describe other methods of data collection.
   Application/NA/Assessment

10. *Correct response: b.* **This is one of ten descriptors discussed in this chapter. It is important for the community system and its resources to be available to all community members.**

Answer choices **a, c,** and **d** describe inappropriate or unhealthy community patterns.

Application/Health Promotion/
Assessment

Aggregates in the Community and Skills of the Community Health Nurse

I. Shifting Care From an Individual Focus
   A. Populations, Aggregates, and Groups as a Unit of Service
   B. Definitions of Terms (Spradley & Allender, 1996)
      1. Population—"A group of people who share one or more environmental or personal characteristics." Example—the homeless population of the United States (they have a location in common), and homelessness (a personal characteristic in common)
      2. Group—"A collection of persons who engage in repeated, face-to-face communication, identify with each other, are interde-

pendent, and share a common purpose." Example—members of a retirement village, swim-club members, student nurses from the same program (a collection of persons who have repeated contact, identify with each other, are interdependent, and share a common purpose)

3. **Aggregate—"A group of people who share some common interest or goal and in community health practice are considered a unified whole in solving problems or promoting health."**

Example—populations and groups are types of aggregates and are the focus of community health care. This is very different from the individual approach in acute care settings. The community health nurse (CHN) uses an aggregate focus when working with populations and groups.

II. The Nurse's Role When Working With Client Groups
A. Advocacy
1. Definition—a process by which the nurse enhances continuity of care through informing, supporting, and affirming clients' self-determination and efficacy in health care decisions

2. **Implementation—speaking or writing on behalf of someone else; using persuasion in support of another**
    a. Taking the initiative to help families
    b. Becoming actively involved in influencing funders to allocate monies for needed services
    c. Identifying available community resources
    d. Assisting clients in pursuing and protecting their legal rights
B. Teaching: process of conveying information to a group by applying educational principles
1. Domains of learning
    a. Cognitive domain: involves the mind and the thinking process; deals with the recall or recognition of knowledge and the development of intellectual abilities and skills
    b. Psychomotor domain: includes visible, demonstrable performance skills that require some kind of neuromuscular coordination
    c. Affective domain: involves emotion, feeling, or affect; deals with interest, attitudes, and values; characterized by attempts to influence clients' values and feelings
2. Teaching and Learning Considerations
    a. *Client readiness:* influenced by many factors including emotional readiness, educational background, maturational level; degree of readiness determines amount of material presented in each teaching session
    b. *Client perceptions:* vary depending on individual but help client interpret and attach meaning to information; vari-

ables influencing perception: values, past experiences, culture, religion, personality, developmental stage, educational and economic level, social forces, and the physical environment

c. *Educational environment:* setting of educational endeavor has a significant impact on learning. Consider the physical environment: lighting, seats, noise, temperature, space, distractions, and so forth. Very important to have an atmosphere of mutual respect and trust. Both the nurse and the learners have a responsibility to establish a mutually satisfying environment.

d. *Client participation:* degree of client participation in the educational process directly influences the amount of learning; contracting (the client participates as a partner to determine goals, content, and time for learning) facilitates learning

e. *Subject relevance to client:* the more relevant the information is to the client, the more readily the subject matter is learned and retained; this is especially true with adult learners who tend to look for the immediate relevance of material taught

f. *Client satisfaction:* client must receive satisfaction from learning to maintain motivation and increase self-direction; obstacles, frustrations and failures discourage and impede learning; realistic goals contribute to client satisfaction

g. *Client application:* learning is reinforced through application, with as many opportunities as possible to apply the learning in daily life

☀ **The role of teacher is one of the most important roles of the CHN.**

3. Group Teaching Methods (Display 5-1)

   a. *Lecture* is used for presenting general information to a

DISPLAY 5-1.
Examples of Teaching Methods

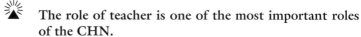

Lecture—explaining the services of an agency to a PTA group

Discussion—in a young mothers' support group, the participants discuss what can be expected from a 2-year-old child

Demonstration—bathing a baby, administering insulin

Return Demonstration—client repeats what was demonstrated

Role Play—a group of teens role play being parents and act out a family discussion regarding allowance or curfew

large group. It is a formal type of presentation and an efficient method of communicating general health information. It creates a passive learning environment due to the limited amount of learner involvement.

    b.   *Discussion* uses two-way communication, which provides the learners with an opportunity to ask questions, make comments, reason out loud, and receive feedback in order to achieve goals; allows participants to learn from each other as well as from the nurse.

    c.   *Demonstration* is used to teach psychomotor skills; is best accompanied by explanation and discussion with time set aside for return demonstrations.

    d.   *Role playing* involves having clients assume and act out roles; start with volunteers and build up to full participation. This technique allows participants to "feel" what it is like to be in another's situation. Discussion should follow guided by carefully prepared questions.

4.   Resources (Materials) for Effective Teaching

    a.   *Materials*—clients have learning enhanced when the teaching also includes pictures, slides, posters, anatomic models, flash cards, chalkboards, videotapes, bulletin boards, pamphlets, flyers, charts and even gestures.

    b.   *Resource acquisition*—the nurse may make the visual aids (posters, slides), buy (anatomic models, videotapes) or acquire them free from companies (eg, videos on infant care from a disposable diaper company, pamphlets on growth and development from an infant formula company) or voluntary agencies such as the American Lung Association, American Heart Association, or the March of Dimes.

C. **Making Home Visits**

   1.   Guidelines for initial contact

    a.   Introduce yourself and the value to the family of the nursing services provided by the agency

    b.   Utilize acute observational skills

    c.   Be sensitive to verbal and nonverbal clues

    d.   Be adaptable and flexible

    e.   Use a "sixth sense" to guide you (trust gut feelings)

    f.   Be aware of your own personality and balance talking and listening

    g.   Remain professional, yet friendly

    h.   Be aware that most clients are not acutely ill and have higher levels of wellness than usually seen in acute care settings

   2.   Guidelines for initial relationship

    a.   Become acquainted with all household members

        b.   Encourage each person to speak for him- or herself

        c.   Be accepting and **listen** carefully

        d.   Help the family focus on issues and move toward desired goals

   3.   Guidelines for ensuring effectiveness

        a.   Be thoroughly prepared by studying the family record, clinic chart, or referral

        b.   Telephone before the visit when possible, introduce self, set a timeframe for the visit

        c.   Physically prepare for the visit; select appropriate literature, information the family will need, and any supplies needed

        d.   Select the most direct route to the home, and approach the home by knocking on the door loud enough to be heard, yet in a friendly manner (don't sound like a bill collector!)

        e.   Spend first few minutes of the visit establishing cordiality and getting acquainted (a mutual discovery or "feeling out" time)

        f.   After the "body" of the visit is over, review the important points, emphasizing family strengths

        g.   Plan with the family for the next home visit

   4.   Guidelines for recording the home visit

        a.   Record the visit in an appropriate manner following agency format

        b.   Complete recording as soon as possible, but certainly before the workday is completed

        c.   Be accurate and complete, fill in all parts, use very brief phrases, remember the family record is **a legal document**

        d.   **Remember, accurate use of records helps to provide continuity of care**

III. **Use of the Nursing Process With Aggregates**

  A. **Assessing Aggregate Needs**

     1.   Collect pertinent data from primary sources (data obtained directly from clients) and secondary sources (data from people who know the aggregate well)

     2.   Analyze and interpret data

  B. **Diagnosing Aggregate Needs**

     1.   Draw up conclusions from interpreted data

     2.   Use the conclusions to develop a nursing diagnosis or problem statement from which planning occurs

  C. **Planning Community Health Programs for Aggregates**

     1.   Follow a logical process of decision making

     2.   Use an orderly and detailed program of action

3. List needs in order of priority
4. Establish goals and objectives of the program
5. Write an action plan with all needed steps through and including an evaluation of the program

D. Implementing the Program or Service

1. Begin to put the plan into action by having all those involved thoroughly prepared
2. Carry out the steps of the plan, modifying individual steps as needed

E. Evaluating the Effectiveness of the Program or Service (The last but a most important phase of the process)

1. **This is an act of appraisal and judging the outcomes of the program or service**
2. **Evaluation measurement is conducted against stated purpose or specific criteria set in the plan**
3. **An evaluation of the performance of those delivering the program and the quality of the program or service itself is also conducted**

IV. The Nurse's Skills When Working With Populations

A. Advocate

1. Advocacy is the art of acting or speaking on behalf of the client
2. The goals of advocacy are to increase client independence and to make a system more responsive and relevant to the needs of clients
3. Special characteristics of advocacy include:
    a. Being assertive
    b. Taking risks
    c. Communicating and negotiating well
    d. Identifying resources and obtaining results

B. Case Manager

1. The case manager exercises administrative direction to accomplish specific goals for a client
2. Goals are achieved through:
    a. Assessing client needs
    b. Planning and organizing to meet the needs
    c. Directing and leading to achieve results
    d. Controlling and evaluating the progress to ensure that goals are met
3. The case manager has to be a decision-maker and have:
    a. Human skills—able to work well with others
    b. Conceptual skills—able to analyze and interpret abstract ideas to meet desired outcomes
    c. Technical skills—able to apply case management knowledge and expertise to effectively serve clients

C. **Clinician**
  1. This is the most familiar CHN role—the provider of care
  2. The nurse ensures health services are provided to individuals, families, groups, and populations
  3. The emphasis of the clinician role is different from basic nursing. It includes:
     a. A holistic focus—the nurse considers the range of interacting systems that affect the collective health of the "client"
     b. A focus on wellness through the promotion of health and the prevention of illness
     c. A bevy of skills expanding the role of the CHN including collaboration with consumers, use of epidemiology and biostatistics, research, leadership in the community and effecting change

D. **Collaborator**
  1. The CHN is a key member of the health care team, making collaboration an essential skill
  2. To collaborate means to work jointly with others in a common endeavor and to cooperate as partners (Spradley & Allender, 1996).
  3. This role requires skills in:
     a. Communication
     b. Interpreting the CHN's role on the health care team
     c. Acting assertively as an equal partner
     d. Functioning as a consultant

E. **Counselor**
  1. An additional skill the CHN must possess is that of listener. The nurse is often in a situation where clients share their most personal concerns. The nurse must know what to do with this information and give appropriate guidance and counseling.
  2. Specific skills the role of counselor requires include:
     a. Active listening
     b. Being open and responsive to clients' needs
     c. Knowing one's own limitations in the counselor role
     d. Knowing the appropriate resources for referral as needed

F. **Educator**
  1. A major function of the CHN is to promote the public's health
  2. Teaches clients at the individual, family, group, or population level
     a. Uses the skills in one-on-one teaching
     b. Uses the skills needed for teaching groups
  3. Aspects about the population served in community health nursing that make the educator role valuable:
     a. The people are not acutely ill and better able to absorb and act on the information

b.   The large numbers of people that can potentially be reached by the CHN give this role importance

G.   Researcher

1.   The role of researcher is to solve problems to enhance community health practice

2.   As a researcher, the CHN engages in:
    a.   Systematic investigation
    b.   Data collection
    c.   Analysis of data

3.   The steps in the research process used by the CHN include:
    a.   Identify an area of interest
    b.   Specify the research question or statement
    c.   Review current literature on the area being studied
    d.   Identify a conceptual framework around which the study will be organized
    e.   Select a research design or method
    f.   Collect and analyze data
    g.   Interpret the results
    h.   Communicate the findings through a presentation, report, or as a nursing journal article

Bibliography

American Nurses Association. (1986). *Standards: Community health nursing practice.* Kansas City, MO: Author.

Brown, M. A. (1988). Health promotion, education, counseling and coordination in primary health care nursing. *Public Health Nursing, 5*(1), 16–23.

Clemen-Stone, S., Eigsti, D. G., & McGuire, S. L. (1991). *Comprehensive family and community health nursing.* (3rd ed.). St. Louis: Mosby–Year Book.

Farley, S. (1993). The community as partner in primary health care. *Nursing and Health Care, 14*(5), 244–249.

Spradley, B. W., & Allender, J. A. (1996). *Community health nursing: Concepts and practice.* (4th ed.). Philadelphia: Lippincott-Raven.

Stanhope, M., & Lancaster, J. (1992). *Community health nursing: Process and practice for promoting health.* (3rd ed.). St. Louis: Mosby–Year Book.

Swanson, J. M., & Albrecht, M. (1993). *Community health nursing: Promoting the health of aggregates.* Philadelphia: W.B. Saunders.

STUDY QUESTIONS

1. A working definition of **group** presented in this chapter is:
   a. "A collection of persons engaged in repeated, face-to-face communication"
   b. "People who share one or more environmental characteristics"
   c. "People who are considered a unified whole in solving problems"
   d. "People who share one or more personal characteristics"

2. When a CHN works as a client advocate, the nurse:
   a. Is aggressive in pursuing the achievement of client goals
   b. Uses a passive approach in solving identified client problems
   c. Is assertive in speaking or writing on behalf of clients
   d. Attempts to smooth problems over to keep the community calm

3. A CHN performs a baby bath demonstration for a class of prenatal parents. This is an example of which of the following domains of learning:
   a. Cognitive
   b. Psychomotor
   c. Affective
   d. Teaching

4. A CHN works with teens in a high school Life Skills class. They are discussing attitudes and feelings about smoking. The nurse uses role playing as a teaching technique. This is an example of which of the following domains of learning:
   a. Cognitive
   b. Psychomotor
   c. Affective
   d. Teaching

5. Client readiness to learn is basic to the teaching/learning process. Which of the following factors influence a client's readiness to learn?
   a. Educational environment
   b. Reinforcing the skills learned

c. Client participation in the educational process
d. Emotional and maturational level of the client

6. An efficient teaching method to present general information to a large group of people is:
   a. Lecture
   b. Discussion
   c. Demonstration
   d. Role playing

7. The CHN leads a class on breastfeeding with a group of prenatal parents. The nurse allows the participants to ask questions, make comments, and reason out loud as feedback is given. The nurse is using which of the following teaching techniques:
   a. Lecture
   b. Discussion
   c. Demonstration
   d. Role playing

8. When beginning a relationship with a family on a home visit, the CHN:
   a. Focuses on the one family member with the "problem"
   b. Encourages others to speak for the main client to get an unbiased view
   c. Is accepting and listens carefully to all family members
   d. Allows the discussion to be open and nondirectional

9. When recording the home visit, it is important for the CHN to:
   a. Complete all charting by Friday, before each weekend
   b. Use complete sentences in a narrative format
   c. Record the visit in a style that is most comfortable and natural for the nurse
   d. Follow the agency format for recording in this legal document

10. One of the roles of the CHN is that of **case manager**. Which of the following best describes that role?
   a. Active listening, giving guidance, knowing one's own limitations, and referrals
   b. Assesses, plans, directs, controls, and evaluates the overall care to clients
   c. Teaches clients, promotes the public's health, works with individuals and groups
   d. Investigates, collects and analyzes data, interprets the results, and shares the findings

ANSWER KEY

1. **Correct response: a**
   Answer choices **b** and **d** are part of the definition for **population**, and answer choice c is part of the definition for **aggregate**.
   Comprehension/NA/NA

2. **Correct response: c**
   Answer choices **a, b,** and **d** describe approaches to be avoided. The nurse needs to remain assertive (supporting clients' rights) and not become either aggressive, passive or attempt to smooth things over. None of these approaches are appropriate.
   Application/Safe Care/Implementation

3. **Correct response: b**
   Answer choice **a** pertains to the mind and the thinking process.
   Answer choice **c** involves the emotion, feeling, or affect.
   Answer choice **d** is the activity that facilitates all three domains of learning.
   Application/Safe Care/Implementation

4. **Correct response: c**
   Answer choice **a** pertains to the mind and the thinking process.
   Answer choice **b** pertains to the visible, demonstrable performance of skills that require some kind of neuromuscular coordination.
   Answer choice **d** is an activity that facilitates all three domains of learning.
   Application/Safe Care/Implementation

5. **Correct response: d**
   Answer choices **a, b,** and **c** are additional components of teaching/learning principles, just as client readiness is one of the principles. Client readiness is determined by emotional readiness, educational background, and maturational level.
   Comprehension/Health Promotion/Assessment

6. **Correct response: a**
   b. Discussion—encourages two-way communication, difficult to do in a large group and not recommended when general information is being shared.
   c. Demonstration—is best conducted with individuals or in small groups with time for the participants to return a demonstration.
   d. Role playing—involves having clients assume and act out roles, again not a technique suited for large groups when transmitting general information.
   Application/Health Promotion/Implementation

7. **Correct response: b**
   a. Lecture—this method is used when presenting general information to a large group. It is formal and efficient with no time for two-way dialogue.
   c. Demonstration—is best conducted with individuals or in small groups with time for the participants to return a demonstration.
   d. Role playing—involves having clients assume and act out roles, again not a technique suited for large groups when transmitting general information.
   Application/Health Promotion/Implementation

8. **Correct response: c**
   Answer choice **a** suggests focusing on one family member. The nurse should give equal attention to all family members to get a better holistic view of the family and perhaps do case finding.
   Answer choice **b** should be discouraged. The nurse should encourage each family member to speak for him- or herself. This is empowering for the individual.
   Answer choice **d** should be limited. Time is important for the nurse and the family, and the nurse needs to keep the

family focused on issues and move toward desired goals.

Application/Health Promotion/ Implementation

9. *Correct response: d. The chart is a legal document and should follow agency format.*

   Answer choice **a**—charting needs to be completed immediately after the home visit or by the end of the workday.

   Answer choices **b** and **c**—the agency format needs to be followed, but rarely is it recorded in narrative with complete sentences or in whatever format the nurse chooses.

Application/Safe Care/Evaluation

10. *Correct response: b*

    Answer choice **a** describes the counselor role.

    Answer choice **c** describes the teacher role.

    Answer choice **d** describes the researcher role.

Comprehension/NA/Implementation

Program Development in the Community: Communication and Collaboration

I. Formulating the Health Program
- A. Begin Planning
- B. Identify the Client Population
- C. Identify Needs
- D. Specify the Size and Distribution
- E. Set Population Boundaries
- F. Clarify Program Perspective
- G. Identify Program Resources

II. Conceptualizing the Health Program
- A. Formulate Ideas
- B. Create Options
- C. Consider Several Solutions

III. Detailing the Health Program Plan
- A. Provide Details
- B. Determine Solution Possibilities
- C. Determine Cost and Resources
- D. Initiate Client Review

IV. Evaluating the Proposed Health Program Plans
- A. Evaluate Solutions
- B. Minimize Options

V. Implementing the Proposed Health Program Plans
- A. Initiate the Plan
- B. Involve the Community

VI. Evaluating the Health Program
- A. Consider the Purpose
- B. Consider the Needs
- C. Consider the Problem
- D. Use the Program Evaluation and Review Technique (PERT)
- E. Use a Gantt Chart

VII. Working in Interdisciplinary Teams in the Community
- A. Collaborate
- B. Seek Out and Value Community Involvement
- C. Motivate and Lead Community Improvement
- D. Transfer Leadership: Letting Go—Knowing When and How

I. Formulating the Health Program

    A. **Begin Planning:** This aspect of planning needs to occur first. Include all people potentially interested in the program, and welcome and consider all ideas.

    B. **Identify the Client Population**

        1. Community

        2. Group

        3. Family

        4. Individuals

    C. **Identify Needs**

        1. Needs of the client population must be identified by both the client group and the health care provider.

        2. **If the client population does not recognize a need for the program, it will not succeed.**

    D. **Specify the Size and Distribution:** The client population must be quantified and must include people:

        1. With the problem

        2. Presently underserved by existing programs

        3. Eligible but not presently using existing programs

    E. **Set Population Boundaries**

        1. How geographically extensive will the program be?

        2. What persons will be eligible for the service?

    F. **Clarify Program Perspective**

        1. Get input from all concerned: providers, administrators, board members, clients, community members and others.

        2. Include data and opinions from those directly and indirectly involved in the program.

    G. **Identify Program Resources**

        1. Complete an assessment of existing resources to support the program and what resources are needed to build the program.

        2. Include personnel, facilities, equipment, and funding amounts.

II. Conceptualizing the Health Program

    A. **Formulate Ideas:** This phase involves formulating ideas and options for solving the identified problem in the community.

    B. **Create Options**

        1. Present and examine each option for its positive and negative aspects.

        2. Focus on options that give the greatest rewards (most apt to meet program goals) with a minimum of risk to the providers and the community.

        3. Use collected data from key people, census information, community forums, surveys of residents in the community, and statistical indicators.

        4.   Involve community members (client population) in this phase of the process.

   C.   **Consider Several Solutions**

        1.   Consider alternative solutions by using a problem-solving board (Table 6-1).

        2.   Make program decisions based on information obtained from the problem-solving board.

III.   **Detailing the Health Program Plan**

   A.   **Provide Details:** This phase involves providing details for each plan so they can be seriously considered by the decision makers.

   B.   **Determine Solution Possibilities**

   C.   **Determine Cost and Resources**

   D.   **Initiate Client Review:** Allow clients the opportunity to review each solution for acceptability. (In Table 6-1, the clients would primarily be the caretakers of elders needing day care, such as adult children and spouses.)

IV.   **Evaluating the Proposed Health Program Plans**

   A.   **Evaluate Solutions:** In this phase, each possible solution is weighted to judge the costs, benefits, and acceptability to the client, community, and providers.

   B.   **Minimize Options:** Only those solutions that will provide the desired outcomes should be considered.

V.   **Implementing the Proposed Health Progam Plans**

   A.   **Initiate the Plan:** In this phase, the best plan is selected to solve the original problem.

TABLE 6-1.
A Problem-Solving Board for an Adult Day Care Center

DESIRED SOLUTION	OPTION ALTERNATIVES	IMPORTANT FACTS	SOLUTION RANKING
Adult Day Care Center	▶ Use a vacant room in the public library at a low cost Mon–Fri	▶ Library may need the room in the future; will have to build a ramp	Third best solution
	▶ Build a freestanding facility	▶ Will take 18 months to build and costs $1,000,000	Best solution
	▶ The Zion Christian Church will donate their activity room Mon–Thurs	▶ Can serve clients only 4 days a week	Second best solution
	▶ Mrs. Riley has two rooms in her home she will donate from 10–2 PM	▶ Timeframe too limited, intrusion on Mrs. Riley, limited parking	Worst solution

B. Involve the Community: The community can support the plan through funding or other efforts. (In Table 6-1, the church's offer is accepted, while the community builds a facility. With this decision, the clients are served immediately, 4 days a week, while the preferred long-term plan of a freestanding building is developed.)

VI. **Evaluating the Health Program: This is a critical phase in the planning process.**
   A. **Consider the Purpose: Is the program fulfilling its purpose?**
   B. **Consider the Needs: Are the client needs for which the program was designed being met?**
   C. **Consider the Problem: Is the problem being solved?**
   D. **Use the Program Evaluation and Review Technique (PERT): This technique is used with large projects.**
      1. Intentions
         a. Focus attention on key developmental parts of the program.
         b. Identify potential program problems.

DISPLAY 6-1.
Gantt Chart—Adult Day Care Center (A simplistic modification of tasks needed to begin operation)

B ---- begin task	**E ---- end task**	**------- duration of task**							
Week	**1**	**2**	**3**	**4**	**5**	**6**	**7**	**8**	**9**
Delegate tasks	B----------------E								
Person A									
Person B									
Person C									
etc.									
Seek church approval	B---------E								
Secure licensing needed	B---E								
Marketing and advertisement	B--								
Secure needed supplies	B--E								
Secure employees	B---E								
Secure volunteers	B--E								
Staff plan curriculum and daily activities						B----------------------------			
Begin planning for a new building							B-------------------		
Physically set up facility							B------E		
Health Department inspection								B---E	
Open facility to the public									B----

      c. Evaluate program progress toward goal attainment.

      d. Provide a prompt, efficient reporting method.

      e. Facilitate decision making.

  2. Three steps

      a. Identify specific program activities.

      b. Identify resources to accomplish these activities.

      c. Determine the sequence of activities for accomplishment.

  3. Design: A flowchart is used with numbers representing three timeframe estimates: optimistic, most likely, and pessimistic.

E. **Use a Gantt chart: This chart specifies timeframe, task, and persons assigned to work on each task. Timeframes are suggested for task allotment intervals (Display 6-1).**

VII. Working in Interdisciplinary Teams in the Community (Table 6-2)

A. **Collaborate: Collaborative efforts between disciplines and agencies are helpful to accomplish program development. Interprofessional collaboration creates:**

  1. A rich mix of talents, skills, and viewpoints

  2. An abundant pool of resources

  3. Much stronger programs

  4. **Community partnerships, networks, and coalitions that can be used to successfully develop the present program**

  5. Alliances for future program development

B. **Seek Out and Value Community Involvement**

  1. **Involve the client population in the planning process.**

  2. Seek out and involve key community members.

  3. Value the client population input—they know their own needs.

TABLE 6-2.
Pitfalls and Keys to Success in Implementing Health Programs

PITFALLS TO SUCCESS	KEYS TO SUCCESS
Inaccurate assessment	Thorough, accurate assessment
Nonvalidation of data with community	Validation of assessment data with community
Lack of community involvement	Involvement of the community
Insufficient resources	Sufficient resources
Lack of coordinated planning	Well-thought-out plan with coordination among team members
Lack of leadership	Good leadership
Poor communication	Open communication
(Smith & Maurer, 1995)	

C.   **Motivate and Lead Community Improvement**

1.   Allow growth of community motivation.
2.   Nourish motivation with encouragement and positive feedback.
3.   Develop skills in community members, by:
   a.   Assigning accomplishable tasks
   b.   Encouraging community members to take on more responsibility within their capabilities

   c.   **Being open to new ideas to individualize the program without changing its purpose and goals (remember this program is for the community members)**
   d.   Beginning to step back as the community assumes more leadership

D.   **Transfer Leadership: Letting Go—Knowing When and How**

1.   Empower the client population to have the necessary leadership skills to continue the program.
2.   Observe community leaders evolve, give assistance when asked for, give input in the form of positive feedback as needed.
3.   Remember, growth takes time (sometimes two steps forward and one step backward). Do not become impatient with the transfer of leadership.

   4.   **Develop leadership skills in the community members so the nurse will not be needed in the future, by:**
   a.   **Becoming less and less direct**
   b.   **Becoming more of a consultant to the community members**
   c.   **Moving on to other community issues and leaving the program in the community members' capable hands**
   d.   **Achieving the program's goals, as the community takes control**

Bibliography

Rakich, J., Longest, B., & Darr, K. (1992). *Managing health services organizations.* (3rd ed.). Baltimore: Health Professions Press.

Roman, D. (1969). The PERT System: An appraisal of program evaluation review technique. In H. Schulberg, A. Sheldon, & F. Baker (Eds.). *Program evaluation in the health fields.* New York: Behavioral Publications.

Smith, C. M., & Maurer, F. A. (1995). *Community health nursing: Theory and practice.* Philadelphia: W. B. Saunders.

Spradley, B. W., & Allender, J. A. (1996). *Community health nursing: Concepts and practice.* (4th ed.). Philadelphia: Lippincott-Raven

Stanhope, M., & Lancaster, J. (1992). *Community health nursing: Process and practice for promoting health.* (3rd ed.). St. Louis: Mosby–Year Book.

STUDY QUESTIONS

1. At the formulation stage of the health program planning process, it is important for the community health nurse to know that:
   a. This is the time to make detailed program decisions
   b. This is the time to consider several solutions to the problem
   c. The client population needs to recognize the need for the program
   d. This is when the geographic and population boundaries are kept open

2. At the detailing phase of the health program planning process, the following steps are followed:
   a. Identify the costs and resources needed for each potential solution
   b. Create several options to explore based on the planning group's desires
   c. Consider several alternative solutions to the problem
   d. Select the best plan to implement in order to meet the need

3. A problem-solving board is used in the health program planning process in order to:
   a. Follow different branches or choices as planning progresses
   b. Graphically display alternative solutions to the problem
   c. Give competing programs an equal chance to be chosen
   d. Guide the planners to when the next step must be taken

4. The community health nurse is using the health program planning process and finds that the group is at a point where the best plan is selected. This is which phase of the process:
   a. Formulation
   b. Conceptualization
   c. Detailing
   d. Implementation

5. Which of the following is true about program evaluation?
   a. Program evaluation is a critical phase in the planning process.
   b. The evaluation is designed and conducted by the clients.
   c. Benefits include a refund of costs from the federal government.
   d. It determines which employees will be hired and fired.

6. The term PERT in health program planning refers to:
   a. The way the nurse and others administer the program being developed
   b. Populations, Environment, Resources and Timing in the planning process
   c. A system called Program Evaluation and Review Technique
   d. A chart used to delineate the timeframe to accomplish the planning steps

7. A Gantt chart is used in health program planning to:
   a. Measure the successes or shortcomings of the program
   b. Map out tasks and persons to do them over a period of time
   c. Identify where the key people are in an organization
   d. Solicit new participants in the health planning process

8. Interdisciplinary collaboration is encouraged in health program planning because it:
   a. Reduces the time needed to accomplish goals
   b. Is a better use of a richer pool of resources
   c. Saves money in the planning and implementation of programs
   d. Helps with licensing and contracts occurring later in the planning

9. The ultimate outcome of the community health nurse's involvement in health program planning should be to:
   a. Stay as involved as possible as a leader throughout the process
   b. Continue to lead the project after implementation to ensure success
   c. Plant the seeds of the idea and step back and let others take control
   d. Develop leadership skills in group members for community control

10. Keys to successful implementation of health programs include:
    a. Open communication
    b. Nonvalidation of data with the community
    c. Insufficient resources
    d. Limited community involvement

ANSWER KEY

1. *Correct response: c*
Answer choices **a** and **b** occur later in the process, in the second (conceptualizing) and third (detailing) phases of the health program planning process, not the first (formulation) phase.

Answer choice **d** is not done. In the formulation phase, geographic and population boundaries are limited and set.
Comprehension/NA/Planning

2. *Correct response: a*
Answer choices **b** and **c** are from the second step of the health program planning process and occur before the detailing phase.

Answer choice **d** is from the implementation phase, a later phase of the process.
Comprehension/NA/Planning

3. *Correct response: b*
The remaining answer choices do not describe any phases or tools used in health program planning.
Comprehension/NA/Planning

4. *Correct response: d*
The remaining answer choices are earlier phases of the process. When one plan is selected, this begins the implementation phase.
Application/NA/Planning

5. *Correct response: a*
In answer choice **b,** the clients may participate in the program evaluation by completing a survey, but they do not design or conduct program evaluations. Answer choice **c** indicates there will be a refund of money from the government. Evaluations do not accomplish this. In fact, there may not be any federal money supporting the plan.

Answer choice **d** may be an outcome of personnel evaluations, or based on staffing needs, but not as an outcome of an evaluation of the program itself.
Comprehension/NA/Planning

6. *Correct response: c*
Answer choices **a** and **b** do not pertain to PERT.

Answer choice **d** describes the Gantt chart used in program planning.
Comprehension/NA/Planning

7. *Correct response: b*
The remaining answer choices have nothing to do with any steps in the health program planning process or the use of Gantt charts.
Comprehension/NA/Planning

8. *Correct response: b*
The remaining answer choices are wrong. Interdisciplinary collaboration has not been proven to save time or money, and it has nothing to do with licensing or contracts.
Comprehension/NA/Planning

9. *Correct response: d*
The remaining answer choices are wrong. They represent what is *not* desired. The nurse should not maintain the leadership role throughout the planning or after implementation, nor does the nurse just plant the seed. Throughout the planning, the nurse works to create leadership skills among the health program planning group members.
Application/NA/Implementation

10. *Correct response: a*
The remaining answer choices are examples of the pitfalls to success.
Comprehension/NA/Planning

Epidemiologic Principles and the Status of Community Health

I.   Definition of Epidemiology
>   **A.**   Greek: comes from three Greek words: *epi*—come down upon, *demos*—the people, *ology*—the study of; the study of that which comes down upon the people
>   **B.**   Modern: the study of the determinants and distribution of health, disease, and injuries in human populations

II.   A Historical Overview of Epidemiology
>   **A.**   Hippocrates: (400 BC) a Greek physician who associated the occurrence of disease with lifestyle and environmental factors
>>   1.   Traced to the roots of epidemiology
>>
>>   2.   Referred to as the first epidemiologist
>
>   **B.**   World Disasters: epidemiology developed as a science as a result of the occurrence of great disasters
>   **C.**   The Crusades: (1000–1500 AD) epidemic and pandemic proportions of diseases killed millions of people
>>   1.   The Black Death alone killed millions in Europe (1345–1348).
>>   2.   England lost one fourth of its population from the plague in 1348.
>>   3.   Other diseases affecting massive groups of people at this time included cholera, bubonic plague, and smallpox.
>
>   **D.**   1800s: the science of modern epidemiology was born. Scientists began to accept, support, and profess the cause-and-effect relationships among host, agent, and environmental factors.
>   **E.**   Florence Nightingale: nursing's roots in epidemiology can be traced to Florence Nightingale (1820–1910)
>>   1.   Nightingale kept detailed records of morbidity and mortality among the military in the Crimean War.
>>   2.   Her statistics, nursing practices, and environmental reform measures reduced the mortality rate, due to disease and infection, from 40% to 2% by the war's end.
>
>   **F.**   1900s: the threat of major epidemic diseases declined and epidemiologists began focusing on other infectious diseases.
>>   1.   The diseases focused on were diphtheria, infant diarrhea, typhoid, tuberculosis, and syphilis.
>>   2.   Data were also beginning to be gathered on the host, agent, and environmental relationships in diseases such as scurvy, cancer, and heart disease.
>
>   **G.**   Present: old and new challenges face epidemiologists today.
>>   1.   Old challenges include cancer, cardiovascular disorders, mental illness, accidents, arthritis, and congenital defects.
>>   2.   New challenges include HIV/AIDS, Ebola, and Dengue Fever (becoming today's "plagues").

III.   Epidemiologic Terminology

    A.   *Morbidity:* relative disease rate; usually expressed as incidence or prevalence of a disease

    B.   *Mortality:* relative death rate; the proportions of deaths at a particular time and place

    C.   *Endemic:* continual presence of a disease or infectious agent in a geographic area

    D.   *Epidemic:* disease occurrence that clearly exceeds normal or expected frequency in a community or region

    E.   *Pandemic:* epidemics that are worldwide in distribution

    F.   *Immunity:* the host's ability to resist disease-causing agents

        1.   Passive: short-term resistance acquired naturally (maternal antibody transfer) or artificially (vaccination that gives temporary resistance)

        2.   Active: longer term resistance (sometimes lifelong) acquired naturally (by infection) or artificially (vaccine inoculation)

 IV.   Epidemiologic Frequency Rates (Display 7-1)

    A.   Incidence: all **new** cases of a disease or health condition appearing during a given time

DISPLAY 7-1.
Incidence and Prevalence Rates/Ratios

The flu has hit Thomas Elementary School. The school nurse reports the following occurrences of the flu for the month of February.

	FEBRUARY 7	FEBRUARY 14	FEBRUARY 21	FEBRUARY 28
Incidence Rate	$\dfrac{12}{400}$	$\dfrac{20}{400}$	$\dfrac{26}{400}$	$\dfrac{19}{400}$

(The incidence is determined for each week. There are 400 children enrolled in this school, and 12 had the flu during the first week in February, 20 during the second, and so forth.

Prevalence Rate	$\dfrac{12}{400}$	$\dfrac{32}{400}$	$\dfrac{58}{400}$	$\dfrac{77}{400}$

(The prevalence rate is determined over the month of February. Among the 400 children enrolled in this school, 77 children had the flu during the month of February— 12 + 20 + 26 + 19 = 77.)

The incidence ratio would be graphically displayed as:

Incidence Ratio	$\dfrac{12}{388}$	$\dfrac{20}{368}$	$\dfrac{26}{342}$	$\dfrac{19}{323}$

Assuming February was the first month any flu cases were reported, the monthly statistics show that, by the end of February, 323 students have not had the flu this year. The ratio is displayed with the number with the condition (numerator) over the number not affected by the condition (denominator).

B.   Prevalence: all cases of a disease or health condition existing in a given population at a given time. The condition may be new or may have affected persons for many years.

C.   Rate: statistical measure with the frequency of an event as the numerator and the number of persons among whom the event occurred as the denominator (Display 7-2)

D.   Ratio: statistical measure in which the numerator is not included in the denominator

V.   **Epidemiologic Models: Tool used to display the multiple factors influencing health and illness in the community. There are three significant models.**

A.   Epidemiologic Triad

1.   The basic model from which others have been developed. (Fig. 7-1)

2.   Its triangular shape incorporates the interaction of three interrelated areas of health and illness.

a.   Host: a human or animal in which infectious agents enter and cause disease. Host factors make the host susceptible. Factors may include age, weight, sex, ethnicity, race, and so forth.

DISPLAY 7-2.
Frequently Used Rates in Epidemiology

RATE CATEGORY	TYPE OF RATE	POPULATION FACTOR
Crude Rate =	$\dfrac{\text{Number of deaths during a year}}{\text{Total (midyear) population}}$	Per 100,000 population
Cause-Specific Rate =	$\dfrac{\text{Number of deaths from a stated cause in a year}}{\text{Total (midyear) population}}$	Per 100,000 population
Age-Specific Rate =	$\dfrac{\text{Number of deaths among persons in a given age group in a year}}{\text{Total (midyear) population of the given age group}}$	Per 100,000 population
Maternal Death Rate =	$\dfrac{\text{Number of maternal (puerperal) deaths in a year}}{\text{Total number of live births in same year}}$	Per 100,000 live births
Infant Death Rate =	$\dfrac{\text{Number of deaths of children} <1 \text{ year of age}}{\text{Total number of live births during the same year}}$	Per 1000 live births
Neonatal Death Rate =	$\dfrac{\text{Number of deaths of infants} <28 \text{ days of age in a year}}{\text{Total number of live births in same year}}$	Per 1000 live births
General Fertility Rate =	$\dfrac{\text{Number of live births during a year}}{\text{Total number of females aged 15–44 at midyear}}$	Per 1000 population

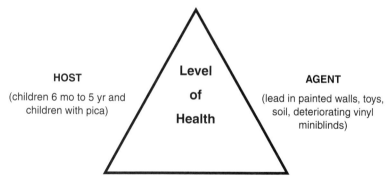

FIGURE 7-1.
The Epidemiologic Triad: Lead poisoning.

b. Agent: the causative factor (present or absent) contributing to a health problem or condition. An example would be the tuberculosis bacteria being *present* and vitamin C being *absent* in scurvy. There are five categories of agents: biologic, chemical, nutrient, physical, and psychological (Display 7-3).

c. Environment: all external factors surrounding the host that might affect vulnerability or resistance. The physical environment includes: geography, climate, weather, safety, water and food supply, and the presence of other organisms that could be reservoirs (storage sites for dis-

DISPLAY 7-3.
Categories of Agents

BIOLOGIC	CHEMICAL	NUTRIENT	PHYSICAL	PSYCHOLOGICAL
Bacteria	Liquids	Essential	Mechanical	Events pro-
Viruses	Solids	dietary	material	ducing stress
Fungi	Gases	components	Atmospheric	
Protozoa	Dusts		Genetically	
Worms	Fumes		transmitted	
Insects				

ease-causing agents) or vectors (carriers for transmitting disease).

B.   Chain of Causation

1.   A more complex way of thinking about disease causation

2.   It identifies where the agent lives and multiplies, how it enters and exits and is transmitted, the agent itself, how it enters the host, and the host itself.

3.   This "chain" is surrounded by the environment, which can influence the outcome at any point (Fig. 7-2).

C.   Web of Causation (Multiple Causation)

1.   This represents the newest and most advanced concept of causation by identifying multiple causative factors.

2.   It is represented by a "web of causation." This web attempts to identify all the possible influences on health and illness.

3.   The web is developed through associated events that lead to a disease process. (The web of causation for myocardial infaction is shown in Fig. 7-3.)

VI.   Epidemiologic Research

A.   The Natural History of a Disease: With all conditions present, the disease or condition follows through its pattern of development. The steps in the natural history of a disease:

1.   Presence of host, agent, and environment

2.   Stage of susceptibility

3.   Stage of presymptomatic (or asymptomatic) disease

4.   Stage of clinical disease

5.   Stage of disability

B.   The Epidemiologic Process in the Community

1.   Determine the natural history of the disease.

2.   Determine the extent of the problem.

    a.   What portion of the population is affected?

    b.   How serious is it to the host?

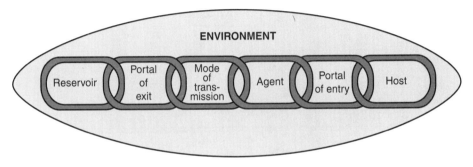

FIGURE 7-2.
Chain of causation in infectious disease.

    c. How is it distributed in the community?

    d. What are the time relationships?

3. Plan a strategy of control.

    a. Identify the vulnerable population.

    b. Where is the agent most vulnerable to attack?

    c. What control measures are available?

    d. What changes in the environment may affect the host favorably?

    e. Set priorities on the basis of relative importance of the problem to the community as a whole.

    f. Develop control measures based on community resources and other factors in the total situation.

4. Establish a control program.

    a. Formulate a workable plan (usually done by those responsible for the situation).

    b. Direct services at prevention, protection, early diagnosis and treatment, limiting disability and rehabilitation.

5. Evaluate the results.

    a. See if objectives were met and compare new situation with the old.

    b. Provide the community with the results, which give a basis for further action.

6. Promote research in order to:

    a. Learn more about the natural history of a health problem

    b. Find improved control measures

    c. Seek better ways to apply control measures

II. Sources of Information for Epidemiologic Study

A. Existing Data

1. Vital statistics

    a. Birth, death, adoption, divorce, and marriage information

    b. Data can be obtained from the local health department.

2. Census data

    a. Population data are collected every 10 years. Estimates are done at 5-year intervals and yearly.

    b. Data can be obtained from national sources available in large libraries.

    c. Analysis of census data provides the community health nurse (CHN) with information about the community. This promotes an understanding of the community and helps to identify specific areas that need further epidemiologic investigation.

3. Reportable diseases

    a. State-developed laws and regulations require health organizations and practitioners to report certain commu-

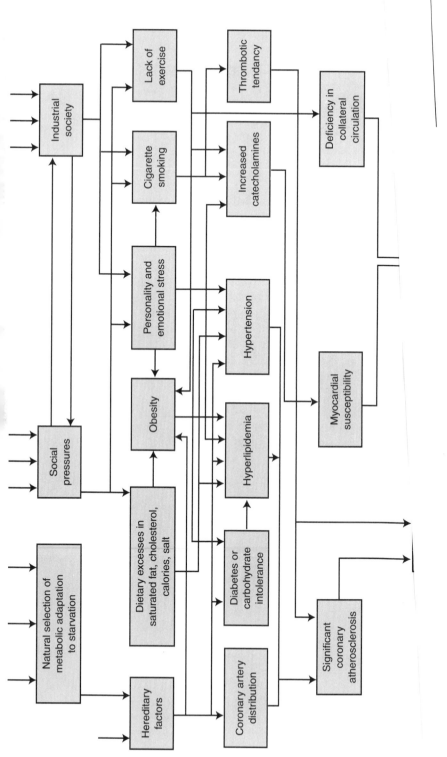

nicable and infectious diseases to the local health authority.
   b. Data can be obtained from the state or local health department.
   c. Follow-up on these diseases is a service provided by health departments through the community health nursing staff.
  4. Disease Registries
   a. Specific disease registries exist in many areas.
   b. The registries provide incidence, prevalence, and survival data for major diseases such as cancer and tuberculosis.
  5. The National Center for Health Statistics (NCHS) Health Surveys
   a. The NCHS provides valuable health prevalence data from surveys they conduct.
   b. 40,000 households are interviewed each year. These surveys provide information about the health status and needs within the country.

B. Informal Investigations
  1. Informal observation is part of the everyday activities of the CHN and often triggers informal study.
  2. Example: The CHN visits several young mothers who have concerns about their toddlers. The CHN asks more mothers about this issue and finds there are many mothers with the same concerns. The CHN starts a class for mothers of toddlers to teach growth and development, provide anticipatory guidance, and answer their questions. The class also serves as a support group for the mothers.

C. Scientific Studies
  1. Carefully designed scientific studies are basic to developing a systematic body of knowledge on which to base nursing practice.
  2. Nurses use the results found in the literature to enhance their practice and positively affect aggregate health.
  3. **Nurses can contribute to this knowledge base by conducting or participating in such studies.**

VIII. Methods of Epidemiologic Investigation
  A. Descriptive
   1. Observes and describes patterns of naturally occurring health-related conditions found in a population
   2. Seeks to establish the occurrence of a problem
   3. Counts the number of occurrences and includes statistical analysis

B. Analytic
    1.   Goes beyond description and observation
    2.   Attempts to identify associations between human diseases, health problems or injuries and their possible cause(s)
    3.   Tests hypotheses or seeks to answer specific questions
    4.   Falls into three categories (in actual practice these types of studies may be mixed)
        a.   Prevalence studies: describe patterns of occurrence by examining causal factors
        b.   Case-control studies: make a comparison between persons with a health problem (the cases) and those without the problem (controls) and look back over time for causative factors in both groups
        c.   Cohort studies: look at a group of people who share a common experience in a specific time period (such groups are called cohorts)

C. Experimental
    1.   Follows and builds on the data gathered from the descriptive and analytic epidemiologic methods
    2.   Occurs under carefully controlled conditions
    3.   Involves one group of subjects who are exposed to some factor (or treatment) thought to cause disease, improve health, prevent disease, or influence health in some way. A second group of subjects are the control group, which has similar characteristics but does not receive the treatment.
    4.   Although experimental studies can be expensive when conducted on a grand national scale and including expensive treatments, the CHN should not overlook opportunities to conduct local experimental studies.

IX. **The Community Health Nurse's Role**
  A. Clinician
    1.   Keep current by reading nursing and public health journals appropriate to the community practice setting
    2.   Use the current literature to enhance practice and improve aggregate health
    3.   Observe the patterns of occurrence and seize opportunities to conduct informal and formal research

  B. Researcher
    1.   Participate in research being conducted by the local community
    2.   Initiate research from observations made in the practice setting
    3.   Follow the steps in conducting epidemiologic research:
        a.   Identify the problem

b. Review the literature

c. Design the study

d. Collect the data

e. Analyze the findings

f. Summarize results and develop conclusions

 g. **Disseminate the findings: this is the most important step. Findings need to be shared with professionals (presentations or journal articles) to strengthen the knowledge base to improve practice and promote future research.**

Bibliography

Berenson, A. S. (1995). *Control of communicable diseases manual* (16th ed.). Washington, DC: American Public Health Association.

Friedman, G. D. (1994). *Primer of epidemiology* (4th ed.). New York: McGraw-Hill.

Lilienfeld, D. E., & Stolley, P. (1994). *Foundations of epidemiology* (3rd ed.). New York: Oxford.

Smith, C. M., & Maurer, F. A. (1995). *Community health nursing: Theory and practice.* Philadelphia: W.B. Saunders.

Spradley, B. W., & Allender, J. A. (1996). *Community health nursing: Concepts and practice.* (4th ed.). Philadelphia: Lippincott-Raven.

Stanhope, M., & Lancaster, J. (1992). *Community health nursing: Process and practice for promoting health.* (3rd ed.). St. Louis: Mosby–Year Book.

STUDY QUESTIONS

1. Principles of epidemiology can be traced back to:
   a. The Crusades
   b. Hippocrates
   c. Florence Nightingale
   d. The Black Death

2. Nursing's roots in epidemiology can be traced to events occurring during the:
   a. Crimean War
   b. Civil War
   c. Late 1800s
   d. Early 1900s

3. In the rural, mountainous area of Madera County, California, there are always three to four cases of plague identified in squirrels. This year, the health department has identified 14 cases of plague in squirrels. This change indicates that this year plague in Madera County is:
   a. Systemic
   b. Endemic
   c. Epidemic
   d. Pandemic

4. So far this winter, the Golden Gate Nursing Center has had 30 residents diagnosed with the flu. During the week of January 5–12, there were 7 cases identified. The flu statistics for this one week are known as the:
   a. Immunity status
   b. Prevalence
   c. Morbidity
   d. Incidence

5. Sally completed the MMR (measles, mumps, and rubella) series and is now protected against these diseases. What type of protection does Sally have?
   a. Natural passive immunity
   b. Artificial active immunity
   c. Artificial passive immunity
   d. Naturally acquired immunity

6. There are 15 members of a weekly hiking group. Six of the 15 (6/15) members got diarrhea from drinking mountain stream water on their last trip. The fraction 6/15 displays which of the following for this trip?
   a. Incidence ratio
   b. Prevalence rate
   c. Incidence rate
   d. Prevalence ratio

7. In the epidemiologic model called the epidemiologic triad, the following aspects are basic to the model:
   a. Host, agent, and environment are placed in a triangular pattern displaying their interrelationship.
   b. All factors that may influence the occurrence of health or illness are identified and displayed in a matrix.
   c. The linking of the disease from its reservoir to entry into the host is displayed in a linear model.
   d. This model focuses on the agent: where it lives, how it multiplies, how it is transmitted, and how it enters the host.

8. In the epidemiologic model called the web of causation, the following aspects are basic to the model:
   a. Host, agent, and environment are placed in a triangular pattern displaying their interrelationship.
   b. All factors that may influence the occurrence of health or illness are identified and displayed in a matrix.
   c. The linking of the disease from its reservoir to entry into the host is displayed in a linear model.
   d. This model focuses on the agent: where it lives, how it multiplies, how it is transmitted, and how it enters the host.

9. When conducting epidemiologic research, the natural history of a disease needs to be identified. This information includes the following:
   a. The progress of the organism from reservoir to the host, giving a historical trail

b. Determining the extent and distribution of the health condition or problem
c. Planning a strategy of control and identifying the vulnerable population
d. With all conditions present, the disease or condition follows its pattern of development

10. The nurses in a local health department are going to conduct an epidemiologic investigation on hepatitis B in their service area. Sources of data that would be most helpful to them would be:
a. Census data
b. Reportable diseases
c. Disease registries
d. The National Center for Health Statistics (NCHS)

ANSWER KEY

1. **Correct response: *b***
   Answer choices **a, c,** and **d** are people and events that contributed to the knowledge level of epidemiology occurring much later than Hippocrates (400 BC), the father of epidemiology.
   Comprehension/NA/NA

2. **Correct response: *a*. During the Crimean War, Florence Nightingale kept statistics on mortality and, through nursing practices and environmental reform, improved the mortality rates significantly.**
   Answer choices **b, c,** and **d** do not represent nursing's roots in epidemiology. Each occurred after the Crimean War. The work done in Crimea influenced the continued focus on epidemiology.
   Comprehension/NA/NA

3. **Correct response: *c*. Epidemic, which means a number that clearly exceeds the normal or expected frequency in a community or region**
   Answer choices **a, b,** and **d** have different definitions not supported by this question.
   Comprehension/Safe Care/Assessment

4. **Correct response: *d*. The statistics from this one week describe the incidence.**
   Answer choice **b** is the prevalence, the accumulated data of the flu in this institution during the winter.
   Answers **a** and **c** are terms in epidemiology but are not related to this situation.
   Analysis/Physiologic/Analysis

5. **Correct response: *b*. Artificial active immunity gives long-term protection through a vaccine. Natural passive immunity occurs through maternal antibody transfer. Artificial passive immunity occurs through a vaccine that gives temporary resistance. Naturally acquired immunity occurs by having the infection.**
   Application/Health Promotion/ Implementation

6. **Correct response: *c*. The question asks about this one trip, so we are looking for incidence (one incident) and it is displayed as a rate, because the total number of people among whom the event occurred is part of the denominator. The other answer choices describe prevalence (all incidents over a stated period) and ratios, where people affected are not included in the denominator (displayed as 6/9).**
   Analysis/Safe Care/Analysis

7. **Correct response: *a***
   Answer choice **b** refers to the web of causation, and choices **c** and **d** refer to the chain of causation.
   Comprehension/Health Promotion/ Analysis

8. **Correct response: *b***
   Answer choice **a** refers to the epidemiologic triad, and choices **c** and **d** refer to the chain of causation.
   Comprehension/Health Promotion/ Analysis

9. **Correct response: *d***
   Answer choice **a** describes the chain of causation.
   Answer choices **b** and **c** are the second and third steps of the epidemiologic process; determining the natural history of a disease is the first step.
   Comprehension/Health Promotion/ Analysis

10. **Correct response: *b*. The nurses can get specific information about this reportable disease in their community.**
    The other answer choices are good resources for information needed when conducting epidemiologic investigations. Census data may be helpful to give all nurses background information for any type of study. It will give information about the population as a whole, age, sex, race, housing, and so forth. Disease registries select specific

disease to focus on, and hepatitis may not be one of them. The NCHS will have information on studies they have conducted and, if they have something on hepatitis, this may be helpful. The most helpful are the statistics on locally reportable diseases.

Application/Safe Care/Implementation

Environmental Influences on Community Health

8

I. A Historical Overview of Environmental Health

   A. Ancient: Environmental issues have influenced people's health throughout history (since the beginning of human existence). Community action to deal with environmental health concerns have been recorded as far back as 2500 BC.

   1. Religious practices protected people's health. For example, the Israelites followed strict rules governing food preparation, sanitation, and quarantining people with infectious diseases, such as leprosy.

2. In Roman, Egyptian, and Indian ruins, thousands of years old, archeologists have uncovered sophisticated water and waste systems.
3. By the Middle Ages, local laws protected city and town dwellers in regard to using river water for washing or selling spoiled foods to local residents.
4. By the 1800s, the cause and effect of some epidemic diseases began to be identified. England led in bringing about environmental changes. Statistics kept and studies conducted by environmental leaders (Edwin Chadwick, Florence Nightingale and John Snow) influenced others in working toward environmental improvement.

B. United States

1. The United States suffered similar environmental "growing pains" as immigration continued, population expanded, and people moved westward.
2. As states organized, some passed specific regulations at the local and state levels to protect residents from diseases and conditions particular to their community or state, such as outlawing "sweatshop" working conditions in immigrant neighborhoods and black and brown lung diseases from mining conditions.
3. National efforts to assess, prevent, and correct environmental health hazards did not become formalized until the 1970s.

II. Causative Factors in Disease, Illness, and Injury

A. Societal Changes

1. Rural ways of living caused catastrophic illnesses when these ways were practiced in the populated areas of towns and cities. (Example: When one family living along a river uses it for drinking water, washing, and disposing of human wastes, the river serves them well. However, when hundreds of families and growing industries use the same river, diseases occur).
2. In the United States and other countries of emigration, immigrant populations crowded into cities of entry and opportunity. Through ignorance and exploitation, their home and work lives were put at risk with unsafe and unhealthy tenement apartment living with long, laborious, and unsafe working conditions.
3. Until the mid-1800s, the professional and scientific community did not know the cause and effect of certain practices. Even now, many lay people do not understand the importance of basic health practices. (Example: A practice as simple as handwashing after toileting needs to be taught to and posted for day care and restaurant employees.)

B. Industrialization Effects

1. Workers: In addition to the problems of a growing number of people coming to the cities, the production processes in which

people were employed put them at risk. Employers did not provide a safe working environment for employees.

2. Pollution: Pollution from the by-products of industrialization, such as particulates in the air, contaminated water supplies, and the esthetics of large industrial operations in communities

C. Causative Agents

1. Chemical
    a. Some substances such as zinc, iron, calcium, and sodium are important to human physiology, but exposure to large amounts can be toxic.
    b. 55,000 natural and synthetic chemicals exist in the United States, 1000 to 1500 are the most hazardous, with only 450 chemicals having been tested for threshold limits.
    c. Exposure to toxic chemicals can cause genetic defects, cancers, and nervous system and brain damage.
    d. Exposure to many hazardous materials occurs in the workplace, either as by-products of or substances used in the manufacturing process.
    e. Exposure may occur at home through peeling lead-based paint, household cleaning products, radon gas buildup, malfunctioning major appliances or heating/cooling systems.
    f. The community health nurses's role includes forestalling or detecting dangers to people at work, school, or home. The ideal intervention comes at the primary prevention level through assessing, teaching, and monitoring .

2. Biologic
    a. Biologic factors are the organisms and potential contaminants found in work, school, and home settings.
    b. These include bacteria, viruses, rickettsias, molds, fungi, parasites, insects, animals, and even toxic plants.
    c. Each biologic agent has the potential to cause an annoying discomfort, a serious disease, or even death.
    d. The community health nurse's role includes teaching about prevention, how diseases caused by bacterial agents are transmitted, and safety around animals of all kinds.

3. Psychological
    a. This category of causative agent responsible for illness or injury in the community is not as obvious as others.
    b. Such elements as noise, overcrowding, traffic, lack of privacy, unavailability of work, lack of safety, fear of potential danger, lack of natural beauty, and boredom can be detrimental to the health of people.
    c. These issues need to be addressed by the community health nurse: at the individual level by teaching anticipatory guidance, healthy coping strategies, and ways of re-

ducing a stressful environment. At the aggregate level the nurse can effect change by being an advocate and leader in contacts with the local and regional government.

    4. Ergonomic

        a. Ergonomics concerns itself with the design of workplaces, tools, and tasks to match the physiologic, anatomic, psychological characteristics and capabilities of workers (Ross, 1994).

        b. More broadly, these concepts apply to school as well as home settings. Comfort and appropriateness of the environment for people of all ages, sizes, and for a variety of purposes are important for well-being.

        c. The community health nurse can assess for environmental effectiveness, and can make suggestions, recommendations, and needed referrals.

III. Social Controls Over Disease, Illness, and Injury

    A. US Legislation

        1. Until the 1970s, there was very little legislation of significance to protect people in the United States against environmental hazards (Display 8-1).

        2. Federal agencies were formed to protect citizens from environmental hazards.

DISPLAY 8-1.
Significant Federal Environmental Legislation

1963	First series of Clean Air Acts
1968	Food and Drug Administration (FDA) became part of the United States Public Health Service (USPHS)
1970	Clean Air Act
1970	Poison Prevention Packaging Act
1970	Occupational Health and Safety Administration (OSHA)
1970	National Institute for Occupational Safety and Health (NIOSH)
1970	Hazardous Materials Transportation Control
1970	National Environmental Policy Act
1971	Environmental Protection Agency (EPA)
1971	Lead-Based Paint Poisoning Prevention Act
1972	Federal Water Pollution Control Act Amendments
1972	Noise Control Act
1976	Resource Conservation and Recovery Act
1976	Toxic Substances Control Act
1977	Clean Water Act
1980	Low Level Radiation Waste Policy Act

B. National Policy

   1. The Public Health Service under the US Department of Health and Human Services developed national health objectives in 1979 and in 1991.

   a. Both documents have an environmental health focus.

   b. The 1991 document has more specific outcome expectations with 22 target areas.

   c. Within each target area are 7 to 22 specific health status objectives, risk reduction objectives, and service and protection objectives.

   2. *Healthy People 2000: National Health Promotion and Disease Prevention Objectives*

   a. This document was developed based on health, illness, and accident statistics observed in the 1980s, with realistic projected expectations for the year 2000.

   b. Sample environmentally focused objectives are listed in Display 8-2.

C. Health Belief Model: widely used since the 1950s to explain wellness and illness behaviors. It has been adapted and tested extensively. The basic premise is that people will take action to avoid disease states.

   1. Actions are motivated by the:

   a. Sense of personal susceptibility to a disease

   b. Perceived severity of a disease

   c. Perceived benefits of preventive health behaviors

   d. Perceived barriers to taking actions to prevent a disease (barriers may include fear, pain, cost, inconvenience, or embarrassment)

   2. Perception of health status and the value placed on taking preventive action may be affected by:

   a. Demographic variables (age, sex, race, ethnicity)

DISPLAY 8-2.
Healthy People 2000—Selected Environmental Objectives

- Reduce the mortality rate among children aged 1–14 years by 15% from 33 to no more than 28 per 100,000.
- Reduce outbreaks of water-borne disease from infectious agents and chemical poisoning to no more than 11 per year.
- Reduce cigarette smoking to a prevalence of no more than 15% among people aged 20 and older.
- Reduce deaths caused by alcohol-related motor vehicle crashes to no more than 8.5 per 100,000.
- Slow the rise in lung cancer deaths to achieve a rate of no more than 42 per 100,000.
- Reduce deaths from work-related injuries to no more than 4 per 100,000 full-time workers.
- Reduce asthma morbidity, as measured by a reduction in asthma hospitalizations to no more than 160 per 100,000.
- Decrease mortality rate of cancer to no more than 130 per 100,000.

        b.   Psychological variables (social class, peer pressure)

        c.   Structural variables (personal experience or knowledge of the disease)

        d.   Internal cues (detecting a breast lump)

        e.   External cues (advice from others and exposure to an educational campaign)

   3.   This model is directed more toward health-protecting behaviors (immunizations, reducing exposure to environmental health hazards) than health-promoting behaviors (fostering personal development or self-actualization). Some behaviors, such as a healthy dietary intake, an exercise routine, and stress management both promote and protect one's health.

D. **PRECEDE Model: "PRECEDE" is an acronym for predisposing, reinforcing, and enabling causes in educational diagnosis and evaluation**

   1.   This health education model uses a problem-solving approach to help groups change behaviors.

   2.   It proposes that health and health behaviors are caused by multiple factors and health education designed to influence behavior must be multidimensional.

   3.   The model has seven phases and is similar to the nursing process (Table 8-1).

E. **Pender's Health Promotion Model: This model attempts to account for those behaviors that improve well-being and develop human potential, which include:**

   1.   Cognitive-perceptual factors: individual perceptions of the importance of health, control over health, and perceived benefits and barriers to health-promoting behaviors

   2.   Modifying factors: demographic, biologic, interpersonal, environmental-situational factors, and learned health-promoting factors and behavior patterns

   3.   Internal and external cues to action

   4.   The above three factors determine a person's likelihood of engaging in health-promoting behaviors.

F. **Human Ecology Model**

   1.   Several human ecology models exist.

   2.   They are based on interrelated biologic and social systems and are similar to the epidemiologic triad but without well-defined separation between host and agent. (See Chap. 7.)

   3.   Sample models include:

        a.   Kulbok's Resource Model of Preventive Health Behavior (1985): proposes that the likelihood of practicing preventive health behaviors increases when more social and health resources are available to the individual.

TABLE 8-1.
Phases of the PRECEDE Model

PHASE	QUESTION	EXAMPLE
Phase I Social diagnosis	What are the group's general concerns?	Sexually active teenagers
Phase II Epidemiologic diagnosis	What are the specific health problems related to the social diagnosis?	Teenage pregnancy, sexually transmitted diseases, (including HIV/AIDS)
Phase III Behavioral diagnosis	What are the health-related behaviors?	Unprotected sexual activity, underage drinking, and illegal drug use
Phase IV Educational diagnosis	What are the predisposing, enabling, and reinforcing factors?	*Predisposing*—peer pressure *Enabling*—drugs, alcohol *Reinforcing*—teen fears rejection by significant other if not engaging in sex, and it is a satisfying activity
Phase V Analysis of educational diagnosis	Which of the priority factors will be focused on during educational plan?	Peer pressure Safety Alternative activities
Phase VI Administrative diagnosis	What specific objectives and resources are needed for the health education plan?	*Objective:* Teens will explore alternative ways to demonstrate caring and love for one another. *Resources:* Community support for teen dialogue, teen health services, and teen-focused, church-sponsored activities.
Phase VII Evaluation	What are the results of the educational plan?	Formation of teen discussion groups, special teen health services at local health department, strengthening of teen church group activities.

Adapted from Green, L., Kreuter, M., Deeds, S., & Partridge, K. (1980). *Health education planning: A diagnostic approach.* Palo Alto, CA: Mayfield Publishing.

b. Shaver (1985): proposes an integrated and holistic human ecologic model of health and wellness with host factors integrated with environmental factors to assess vulnerability, risk, and personal response to actual or potential health needs.

IV. Present Environmental Areas of Concern

A. Water Pollution

 1. **Water in adequate quantity and purity is essential to the health of a society for consumption, as a medium for the survival of plants and animals, carrying and distributing necessary nutrients in the environment, and recreation.**

2. Two main sources are:
a. Surface water from lakes and streams
b. Groundwater found underground in aquifers, coming to the surface through springs and wells

3. Contamination occurs in three ways:
a. Infection with bacteria, parasites or viruses can cause diseases if the water is not treated before consumption.

 (Even crystal clear water from mountain streams can carry *Giardia lamblia*, a parasite from human and animal wastes, which causes giardiasis, an intestinal disease resulting in diarrhea and malabsorption of nutrients.)

b. Toxic substances are introduced by humans usually through farming pesticides, oil spills, personal and industrial dumping, and burying hazardous wastes. Over time, they seep into the groundwater or pollute lakes and streams.
c. Heat introduced into lakes and streams by industry, namely nuclear power plants, causes water temperatures to rise and negatively affects beneficial organisms in the water.

B. Air Pollution

1. For centuries, people have been aware of the negative effects of poor air quality. Thousands of deaths have been reported due to episodes of concentrated pollutants in the environment due to thermal atmospheric inversions. (Historically in London and in other metropolitan areas, many people died due to trapped pollutants in the atmosphere.)

 2. **Air pollution is recognized as one of the most hazardous sources of chemical contamination. (Radon gas buildup is air pollution in the home.)**

 3. **Most air pollution results from industrial and automotive emissions, including lead, ozone, carbon monoxide, sulfur dioxide, hydrocarbons, nitrogen oxides, and particulates such as ash and dust.**

4. Airborne pollutants have many negative effects on human life including costs to property, productivity, quality of life, and human health.

5. Diseases and symptoms associated with specific air pollutants range from minor nose and throat irritations, respiratory infections, and bronchial asthma, emphysema, cardiovascular disease, lung cancer, and genetic mutations.

6. In addition to negative effects on humans, air pollution upsets the ecosystem.
   a. "Acid rain": air pollutants and nitrogen oxides combine with water vapor and cover the earth with toxins.
   b. "Greenhouse effect": carbon dioxide buildup traps infrared heat near the earth's surface and raises the earth's temperature, affecting normal flora and fauna.

C. Unhealthy or Contaminated Food: There are three categories of hazardous foods.

1. Inherently harmful
   a. Poisonous foods (some mushrooms and berries) and harmful plants (oleander) are examples of items that cause illness or death if consumed.
   b. People need to know what poisonous or toxic plants are growing around their home or are found in nature and to avoid them. This is especially important for children.

2. Contaminated

   a. **Contaminated food is a growing public health problem and is related to inadequate processing, handling, storing, and shipping methods.**
   b. Increased number of outbreaks of harmful bacteria such as *Salmonella, Staphylococcus, Escherichia coli,* and *Clostridium* are occurring.
   c. Other contaminants include parasites, worms, and chemicals. Chemical contamination comes from dirty processing machinery, pesticides, and herbicides. Mercury has been found in fish from polluted water and has caused severe neurologic damage and death. It is rare that foods are contaminated with viruses.
   d. Public health guidelines reinforce appropriate handling and storing and cooking meats thoroughly. Recent shocking reports of deaths, in otherwise healthy people, have been traced back to eating undercooked contaminated beef in fast-food restaurants.

3. Toxic additives
   a. Food additives enhance the preservation, flavor, and color of foods, making them more marketable and appealing. Many of the chemicals used have the potential to be toxic.

(Red dye #2 and saccharin, once liberally used, have been found to be hazardous and have been removed from foods.)

b. Other additives in use, such as NutraSweet, may have long-term effects not yet known.

c. Added salts and sugars, although they are not considered "toxic" by most people, are not recommended in a health conscious diet.

D.   Human and Hazardous Waste Disposal

1. 1000 to 1500 pounds of solid waste products are produced by each person every year in addition to 2000 pounds produced by industry per person each year.

2. Methods of waste disposal are limited, and none is ideal.
   a. Burning (transforming it into another pollutant)
   b. Hiding (storing in metal canisters, vacant lots filled with old auto tires, and so forth)
   c. Burying (in landfills that in time have the potential to decompose and seep toxic substances into groundwater if not treated properly)

3. Sanitary landfills treat the waste products, seal them to avoid rodent infestation and water stagnation, and have proven to be a satisfactory way of dealing with nontoxic solid wastes.

4. Hazardous waste disposal is an important issue. Toxic chemicals, radioactive wastes, and infectious wastes are presently being buried in landfills in double-lined cells.

5. Over time and among less reputable waste control companies, the system may break down or not be followed, thus creating risks now and for future generations.

E.   Insect and Rodent Control

1. Insect and rodent control is a worldwide problem. Insects and rodents:
   a. Are nuisances
   b. Cause economic damage
   c. Are links (vectors) in the chain of causation in disease transmission

2. Common vectors are mosquitoes, flies, ticks, roaches, fleas, rats, mice, and ground squirrels and are known to transmit scores of diseases.

3. The methods of control are focused at the primary and secondary level of prevention and include:
   a. Primary level: eliminate breeding sites and improve sanitary conditions
   b. Secondary level: trap rodents, poison, and spray with pesticides

F. **Safety at Home, the Worksite, and the Community: people can be exposed to toxic chemicals, radiation, injury, and psychological hazards in the activities of daily living.**

    1. Toxic chemicals

        a. Home/garage: in household products used for cleaning, protecting, and repairing

        b. Work: in varying amounts depending on the company and its activities

        c. Community: in keeping up community lawn areas or spraying for mosquitoes

    2. Radiation occurs naturally in the environment from the sun, soil, and minerals.

        a. Homes: in electronic devices such as television sets and microwave ovens

        b. Work, health centers or health care provider offices: in some manufacturing processes, lasers and radiographs

    3. Injury: primary prevention of injury should be the focus of people at home, work, or in the community

        a. Home: providing a safe home environment

        b. Work: following safety guidelines and using protective devices

        c. Community: driving safely using proper restraints. Always think of *safety* first, in spite of convenience and, at times, comfort.

    4. Psychological hazards exist within home, work, and community environments and affect feelings of well-being. They should not be overlooked (see Section II: C:3).

V. **The Nursing Process and Environmental Health (Display 8-3)**

  A. Assessment

    1. Produce data that will help determine an environmental health diagnosis.

    2. Begin locally in the homes and neighborhoods of clients and move out to the broader community.

    3. Assess for potential environmental hazards to avert occurrences at the primary level of prevention.

  B. **Diagnosis: made from all the data collected. This will give direction for action in the next phase of the process.**

  C. Planning

    1. Formulate a plan of action to prevent, ameliorate, or remove/stop the environmental health problem. (The plan may be as simple as making a referral to the appropriate agency and following through on action taken or as complex as lobbying legislators at state and national levels to change state or national environmental health laws.)

DISPLAY 8-3.
Use of Nursing Process With an Environmental Health Issue

RODENT AND INSECT INFESTATION IN A PUBLIC HOUSING DEVELOPMENT

Gather data about the reported problem by speaking with clients, maintenance, and the apartment manager.

Assessment

Assess the extent of the problem (six families involved), who is involved (families on two floors in one section of the building), what type of problem they are having (rats, cockroaches, ants), what have the clients done to prevent or control the problem (four families keep food in kitchen only, pet food off the floor after they eat, dishes washed daily, but two families have food left out in all rooms of the apartment, wash dishes sporadically, have pet food on the floor, have three indoor pets, and they live on the first floor), how has the management responded (sent exterminators, but the two families with unsafe practices refused to let them in).

Diagnosis

Make a nursing diagnosis from the gathered data:

Insect and rodent infestation in six apartments related to unsanitary living conditions of two families in adjoining apartments.

Reinforce manager's infestation elimination efforts in the four apartments being affected by the offending residents.

Planning

Make a shared home visit with the Department of Health environmentalist to discuss the situation with each family.

Take needed interventions.

Monitor results.

Implementation

Home visit to two offending families—both families were initially unreceptive but allowed the home visit. Inquired into their perception of the problem—"dogs are for our safety and bugs don't bother us." Take needed interventions—teach reasons to be concerned, such as health and safety of their children and pets, effects on other residents, aesthetics, and the risk of eviction. Determine methods of control they will comply with. They agreed to clean up daily, try to limit eating to one or two rooms, feed dogs once a day and clean up the pet area after eating.

Monitor results—follow-up visits by nurse and environmentalist weekly for 3 weeks to assess for changes and to reinforce positive efforts to make change.

Evaluation

Compare the problem now with the initial problem. Three affected families have no problem. With one family, the infestation with cockroaches continues but is not as bad. The two offending families have made significant changes, as observed on the three follow-up visits. However, one of these families has gotten two more dogs, and the manager will begin eviction proceedings if they don't limit indoor pets to two, as stated in their lease.

Based on the follow-up visits, one family will have two more visits and a visit will be made to the one affected family still experiencing some infestation. They may have changed some practices.

    2. Recognize the nurse's role in improving health at the environmental level (often done in interdisciplinary teams). This may be a new concept for many nurses and needs to be emphasized.

D. Implementation

    1. Act or implement the designed plan.

    2. Use an interdisciplinary approach to accomplish change and solve problems. This interdisciplinary approach to environmental health problems is critical in the planning and implementation phases.

E. Evaluation: an important phase of the process that must not be overlooked

    1. Review the objectives of the plan to see if the outcomes expected have actually been accomplished.

    2. Modify the assessment, planning or implementation phase in order to have more precise outcomes. This must be discovered during the evaluation phase.

    3. Continue with additional action after the evaluation is complete.

VI. The Nurse's Role in Promoting Environmental Health

    A. Observe: Use the nursing process with individuals, families, groups, and aggregates to observe for incidences of illness or injury and to prevent or eliminate an environmental health hazard.

    B. Educate: Teach individuals and groups how to live a healthy and safe lifestyle and how and where to report any environmental hazards they may observe.

    C. Advocate: Be a client advocate and report any incidents of potential or existing environmental hazards.

    D. Collaborate: Collaborate with interdisciplinary team members and enter into partnerships in the community to prevent potential problems and to solve identified environmental health problems.

    E. Research: Keep knowledgeable and informed about current environmental legislation, local law changes, and new environmental hazards occurring locally, regionally, or nationally so you can be a source of information to professionals and clients in the community.

Bibliography

Green, L., Kreuter, M., Deeds, S., & Partridge, K. (1980). *Health education planning: A diagnostic approach*. Palo Alto, CA: Mayfield Publishing.

Kulbok, P. (1985). Social resources, health resources, and preventive health behavior: Patterns and predictions. *Public Health Nursing, 2*(2), 67–81.

Last, J. M. (1987). *Public health and human ecology*. East Norwalk, CT: Appleton and Lange.

Moeller, D. W. (1992). *Environmental health*. Cambridge, MA: Harvard University Press.

Pickett, G., & Hanlon, J. (1990). *Public health: Administration and practice* (9th ed.). St. Louis: Times-Mirror/Mosby.

Ross, P. (1994). Ergonomic hazards in the workplace: Assessment and prevention. *AAOHN Journal, 42*(4), 171–176.

Shaver, J. (1985). A biopsychosocial view of human health. *Nursing Outlook, 33*(4), 186–191.

Smith, C. M., & Maurer, F. A. (1995). *Community health nursing: Theory and practice.* Philadelphia: W.B. Saunders.

Spradley, B. W., & Allender, J. A. (1996). *Community health nursing: Concepts and practice.* (4th ed.). Philadelphia: Lippincott-Raven.

Swanson, J. M., & Albrecht, M. (1993). *Community health nursing: Promoting the health of aggregates.* Philadelphia: W.B. Saunders.

US Department of Health and Human Services. (1991). *Healthy people 2000: National health promotion and disease prevention objectives.* Washington, DC: Government Printing Office.

STUDY QUESTIONS

1. It has been found that in ancient societies environmental health was of concern to the people by the discovery of:
   a. Healthy-appearing skeletons found in unearthed graves
   b. Sophisticated water and waste systems
   c. Recently found writings describing environmental practices
   d. Pottery with pictures on them depicting health statistics

2. In the 1800s, positive growth of an environmental health movement in the United States was thwarted by:
   a. Urban growth, westward movement, and an independent spirit
   b. The complexities of the changing terrain in such a large country
   c. Weather conditions not previously experienced by the immigrant citizens
   d. Political, religious, and economic issues of the times

3. An example of a biologic causative agent affecting the environment is:
   a. Household cleaning agents
   b. Population overcrowding
   c. Toxic plants
   d. The shape and structure of office furniture

4. Significant legislation regarding environmental health seriously began in the:
   a. 1890s
   b. 1920s
   c. 1950s
   d. 1970s

5. In the document *Healthy People 2000,* one will find:
   a. National health promotion and disease prevention objectives
   b. Lists of diseases, illnesses, and accidents affecting people
   c. Ways and means to keep all people healthy
   d. Profiles of what a healthy person in the United States looks like

6. The purpose of the PRECEDE Model is to:
   a. Develop an epidemiologic approach to health education
   b. Account for behaviors that improve well-being and develop human potential
   c. Direct a health education model toward health-protecting behaviors
   d. Present a health education model that uses the problem-solving approach

7. A safe water supply is basic to environmental health. Sources of water pollution are:
   a. Cosmic energy that occurs naturally in the atmosphere
   b. Infective substances such as bacteria and parasites
   c. Surface water that seeps into the groundwater
   d. Groundwater coming to the surface through wells and springs

8. Air pollution is a serious environmental health issue. The following is true about air pollution:
   a. It is a recent phenomenon, coming about since the 1950s.
   b. It is one of the most hazardous sources of biologic contamination.
   c. It results from industrial and automotive emissions.
   d. It has been a major problem since the beginning of mankind.

9. Waste disposal in the United States is of environmental concern because:
   a. Nontoxic landfills, even treated properly, are unsatisfactory methods of handling solid wastes
   b. The ideal treatment of waste products is to hide them, and we are running out of hiding places
   c. Burning wastes is our only effective way of handling waste disposal

    d. More than 1 1/2 tons of wastes are produced yearly by each person in the United States

10. When solving environmental health problems, the community health nurse seeks out the extent of the problem, questions all people involved, and formulates a nursing diagnosis. This describes which phase of the nursing process:

    a. Assessment

    b. Planning

    c. Implementation

    d. Evaluation

ANSWER KEY

1. *Correct response: b*
Answers **a** and **d** are incorrect responses. Answer choice **c** is also incorrect in that there have not been *recent* findings of writings to indicate environmental efforts. The Bible and other ancient writings found long ago indicate environmental concerns.
Comprehension/Safe Care/Analysis

2. *Correct response: a*
Situations in the remaining answer choices may have existed in the 1800s, but the situations depicted in answer **a** affected the environmental health movement more significantly.
Analysis/Health Promotion/Analysis

3. *Correct response: c*
The other answer choices are examples of chemical, psychological, and ergonomic factors, respectively.
Comprehension/Safe Care/Assessment

4. *Correct response: d*
Significant legislation began in the 1970s, with over 13 acts passed or environmentally focused agencies formed. In the decades before 1970, little environmental legislation occurred.
Knowledge/Safe Care/NA

5. *Correct response: a*
The remaining answer choices are incorrect. *Healthy People 2000* identifies national objectives we should achieve by the year 2000 in major disease and injury areas affecting people in the United States. It gives the numbers of occurrences during key years in the 1980s and projects acceptable numbers of occurrences by the year 2000.
Comprehension/Health Promotion/Assessment

6. *Correct response: d*
Answer choice **a** describes a human ecology health education model. Answer choice **b** describes Pender's Health Promotion Model, and choice **c** describes the Health Belief Model.
Comprehension/Health Promotion/NA

7. *Correct response: b*
Answer choice **a** is incorrect. Cosmic energy does not pollute water supplies.
Answer choice **c** can only pollute the water supply if either water source has been exposed to pollutants. Mixing surface and groundwater does not cause pollution. Answer choice **d** is a description of how groundwater gets to the surface for use.
Comprehension/Safe Care/Analysis

8. *Correct response: c*
Answer choice **a** is incorrect. Air pollution has been a major problem since industrialization.
Answer choice **b** is incorrect. Air pollution is hazardous due to chemical contamination.
Answer choice **d** is incorrect because it was not a major problem until the Industrial Age. However, smoke-filled caves could have polluted the air cave dwellers inhaled.
Comprehension/Safe Care/Analysis

9. *Correct response: d*
Answer choice **a** is incorrect. A landfill is a satisfactory method of handling solid nontoxic wastes.
Answer choice **b** is incorrect. Hiding solid waste does not solve the problem.
Answer choice **c** is incorrect. Burning solid waste transforms it into another pollutant.
Comprehension/Safe Care/Analysis

10. *Correct response: a*
The examples are from the first phase of the nursing process, assessment. The other answer choices are incorrect.
Comprehension/NA/NA

Unit III
Community Health Nursing: Principles of Practice

A Theoretical Basis to Community Health Nursing

I. Theory

A. Broad Definitions

1. "A clearly stated, operationally defined set of concepts, statements, and hypotheses. A collection of principles and rules." (Stanhope & Lancaster, 1992)
2. "A theory is a set of systematically interrelated concepts or hypotheses that seek to explain and predict phenomena." (Spradley & Allender, 1996)

B. Nursing-Specific Definitions

1. "Theory organizes the relationships between the complex events that occur in a nursing situation so that we can assist

human beings. Simply stated, theory provides a way of thinking about and looking at the world around us." (Torres, 1986)

2. "A statement that purports to account or characterize some phenomena. A nursing theory, therefore, attempts to describe or explain the phenomenon called nursing." (Barnum, 1990)

II.   The Value of a Theoretical Base to Practice

A.   Basic Nursing Practice

1. A theoretical basis to practice helps nurses in all settings understand:
   a. Human beings
   b. Health and illness
   c. Problem solving
   d. Creative processes
   e. Human–environment relationship
2. Knowledge of these concepts comes from:
   a. Personal experience
   b. Logic
   c. Ethics
   d. Empirical science
   e. Aesthetic preferences
   f. An understanding of what it means to be human

B.   Community Health Nursing

1. A theoretical basis to community health nursing practice guides nurses on issues such as:
   a. Inequitable health care access
   b. The effects of poverty
   c. Destruction of the environment
2. Knowledge of these issues helps the nurse to bring about changes that:
   a. Positively affect the health of individuals, families, and groups
   b. Promote health
   c. Prevent disease
   d. Maintain levels of wellness

III.   Theories Most Applicable to Community Health Nursing

A.   Public Health Theory

1. Description: Public health theory is concerned with the health of populations of human beings (Smith & Maurer, 1995). It evolves from Winslow's classic definition of public health (see Chap. 1), values cooperation and collaboration, and serves all people for the greater benefit of society as a whole.
2. Significant theorist: C. E. A. Winslow, 1920 (Pickett & Hanlon, 1990)
3. Application
   a. Integrates public health principles and values with basic nursing care

      b. Focuses on reaching people where they live, work, and play

      c. Includes holistic and interdisciplinary services (needs in the community overlap many disciplines)

      d. Collaborates with multiple subsystems

B. General Systems Theory

    1. Description: general systems theory states that every living system is a whole and its wholeness is made up of interdependent parts in interaction (von Bertanlanffy, 1968). This theory provides the foundation to understand how communities function as living systems.

    2. Significant nursing theorist: Neuman, 1989

    3. Application

      a. Addresses many sizes of systems: individuals, families, groups, large aggregates, populations

      b. Deals with open systems (systems that exchange matter, energy, and information with the environment) that have identified boundaries; assesses and seeks to facilitate their client systems' ability to maintain their boundaries and engage in healthy exchanges with their environment

      c. Organizes people (smaller systems) into larger systems, such as the health care system, legal system, educational system (each being a subsystem of a larger system of neighborhood, town, city, state, country, continent, hemisphere, world, and universe)

      d. Increases stability and adaptability of systems; allows an increase in adaptability as a system grows and learns (rapid and significant change can lead to instability and functional disruption, such as in a family dealing with the death of a child or a community rebuilding after a devastating tornado)

      e. Generalizes universal information about individuals, families, and groups as systems to increase effectiveness in working with larger community systems

C. Adaptation Theory

    1. Description: This theory draws from systems theory and recognizes that systems are adaptive. Each system responds to stimuli and initiates control processes to deal with different stimuli through the use of coping mechanisms. Healthy coping promotes growth and is adaptive, whereas unhealthy coping is maladaptive. Adaptation levels constantly fluctuate in systems and direct overall functioning.

    2. Significant nursing theorists: Roy, 1976; Roy & Roberts, 1981; based on Hans Seyle's work on stress, 1956

3. Application
   a. Forms a basis for understanding how human systems function
   b. Provides a means for assessing client's coping abilities
   c. Enables designing nursing actions to facilitate positive adaptation

D. Self-Care Theory

1. Description: This theory has been classified as a systems model and more recently as a developmental model. Self-care consists of those activities that a person does for him- or herself to maintain life, health, and well-being. If the self-care demand is greater than the ability of the person (self-care agency) providing the care, then there is a self-care deficit. When there is a deficit, nursing intervention is facilitated to eliminate it.

2. Significant nursing theorist: Orem, 1985

3. Application
   a. Identifies the self-care ability of the client to develop an appropriate plan of action (a person who wants to quit smoking, a group who needs infant care information, or community agencies planning a health fair)
   b. **Focuses on increasing the self-care abilities of the client**
   c. Develops the skills, knowledge, attitudes, and resources needed for self-care
   d. Works toward reducing the self-care deficit and restoring the self-care agency to the client

E. Science of Unitary Human Beings

1. Description: This theory has strong ties to general systems theory and has four components: energy fields, universe of open systems, pattern and organization, and four-dimensionality. The emphasis is on energy fields as a part of a person's wholeness and the four-dimensionality transcending the time–space interaction. Unitary persons are developed through the use of three principles of hemodynamics: helicy, resonancy, and complementarity. This theory has had an impact on nursing curricula and research projects and is more recently beginning to guide nursing practice, especially among nurses who practice holistic nursing and therapeutic touch (Krieger, 1981). Limitations to this theory include difficult terminology and unclear operational application in the practice setting.

2. Significant nursing theorist: Rogers, 1970; 1989

3. Application (Display 9-1)
   a. Focuses on wholeness of the client system and considers all other systems interacting with the client
   b. Assesses the levels of wellness in the client and works toward improving the wellness level

DISPLAY 9-1.
Application of the Science of Unitary Human Beings

A WEEKEND JOGGER

One community health nurse may praise a client for being physically active and remind him or her about safety. The nurse using Roger's nursing theory considers the wholeness of the client system, four-dimensionality, and system openness. The client's interest in jogging is used to approach caregiving in the following manner:

Activity—changes physical activity to exercise throughout the week and explores other enjoyable activities

Safety—watches traffic, wears appropriate clothing, varies jogging with other forms of exercise to use all muscle groups, avoids high pollution routes, and transfers safety consciousness to other aspects of life

Religion—uses solo exercise time to reflect on the meaning of life and his or her place in the universe and uses this enlightenment to enrich his or her own life and the lives of others

Nutrition and hydration—eats a well-balanced diet rich in nutrients, increases fluids before and after exercising, and uses this information with others he or she is responsible for

Sleep and rest—balances activity with healthy sleep habits and adequate rest and relaxation, sharing these principles with others

Health promotion—follows routine health care parameters incorporating concepts from holistic health care and other disciplines in addition to Western medical practices; remains open to new health promotion ideas for self and others

---

  c. Integrates the concept of open systems in the practice
  d. Transcends time and space to reach a plane of existence (to overcome pain). The Rogerian nurse encourages this belief system for many people.
F. Adult Learning Theory
  1. Description: It is the contention of this theory that learning is an internal process involving the person intellectually, emotionally, and physiologically. A critical part of adult learning is interacting with the environment. Thus, a critical function of the teacher (community health nurse) is to create an environment that allows numerous options for adult students. This theory takes into consideration the independent, self-directed adult with an accumulation of life experiences, and a developmental readiness to learn.
  2. Significant theorist: Knowles, 1980
  3. Application
   a. Teaches adult clients differently than children
   b. Builds on the adult student's experiences to apply new learning identified by the adult client
   c. Adapts learning activities to the relevancy for each client
   d. Acts as a co-leader and co-learner in the educational process
   e. Incorporates self-evaluation of personally developed criteria (this is superior to teacher evaluation of imposed criteria)

Bibliography

Barnum, B. S. J. (1990). *Nursing theory: Analysis, application, evaluation*. Glenview, IL: Scott, Foresman/Little Brown Higher Education.

Knowles, M. (1980). *The modern practice of adult education: From pedagogy to andragogy*. Englewood Cliffs, NJ: Prentice-Hall.

Krieger, D. (1981). *Foundations for holistic health nursing practices: The renaissance nurse*. Philadelphia: J.B. Lippincott.

Marriner-Tomey, A. (1989). *Nursing theorists and their work* (2nd ed.). St. Louis: Mosby–Year Book.

Neuman, B. (1989). *The Neuman systems model, application to education and practice* (2nd ed.). Norwalk, CT: Appleton-Lange.

Orem, D. (1985). *Nursing: Concepts of practice* (3rd ed.). New York: McGraw-Hill.

Pickett, G. E. & Hanlon, J. J. (1990). *Public health administration and practice* (9th ed.). St. Louis: Times Mirror/Mosby.

Rogers, M. E. (1970). *An introduction to the theoretical basis of nursing*. Philadelphia: F.A. Davis.

Rogers, M. E. (1989). Rogers' science of unitary human beings, In Parse, R. R. (Ed.). *Nursing science. Major metaparadigms, theories, and critique*. Philadelphia: W.B. Saunders, pp. 139–146.

Roy, C. (1976). *Introduction to nursing: An adaptation model*. Englewood Cliffs, NJ: Prentice-Hall.

Roy, C., & Roberts, S. L. (1981). *Theory construction in nursing: An adaptation model*. Englewood Cliffs, NJ: Prentice-Hall.

Selye, H. (1956). *The stress of life*. New York: McGraw-Hill.

Smith, C. M., & Maurer, F. A. (1995). *Community health nursing: Theory and practice*. Philadelphia: W.B. Saunders.

Spradley, B. W., & Allender, J. A. (1996). *Community health nursing: Concepts and practice*. Philadelphia: Lippincott-Raven.

Stanhope, M. & Lancaster, J. (1992). *Community health nursing: Process and practice for promoting health*. (3rd ed.). St. Louis: Mosby–Year Book.

Torres, G. (1986). *Theoretical foundations of nursing*. Norwalk, CT: Appleton-Century-Crofts.

von Bertanlanffy, L. (1968). General systems theory: A critical review. In Buckley, W. (Ed.). *Modern systems research for the behavioral scientist*. Chicago: Aldine.

STUDY QUESTIONS

1. A theory can be defined as:
   a. Flexible and disassociated ideas guiding decision making
   b. A set of systematically interrelated concepts or hypotheses
   c. An idea based on experience, whether supported by data or not
   d. A way of looking at and changing some phenomenon

2. A nursing theory is used in an attempt to:
   a. Control the lives of clients who need the external guidance
   b. Organize the work day in order to accomplish all activities
   c. Describe or explain the phenomenon called nursing
   d. Provide a way of conducting nursing practice

3. The value of nursing theory to community health nursing includes:
   a. Guiding practice in the complex community setting
   b. Viewing poverty through the eyes of community members
   c. Equalizing health care access in the community
   d. Eliminating destruction of the environment

4. Public health theory and basic nursing comprise community health nursing, which is distinguished by:
   a. A focus on tertiary levels of prevention among community members
   b. Blending the best of both to create a new specialty in nursing
   c. Providing interdisciplinary services to promote health in communities
   d. Directing care to those who can afford it so services can continue

5. A theorist who bases a nursing theory on the General Systems Theory is:
   a. Rogers
   b. Orem
   c. Knowles
   d. Neuman

6. An open system can be described as a system that:
   a. Exchanges matter, energy, and information with its environment
   b. Substitutes being static for being adaptive
   c. Is in chaos and experiencing functional disruption
   d. Is naturally limited in the universe and hard to achieve on earth

7. An example of a client's behavior that demonstrates the constructs of the adaptation theory includes a:
   a. Gang member who continues the gang lifestyle after giving birth
   b. Widow of 1 year who continues to set the table for her deceased husband
   c. Pregnant teen who is taking childbirth education classes after school
   d. Once-active woman, now wheelchair bound, stays in her home all the time

8. An example of a client's behavior that demonstrates the constructs of the self-care theory includes a diabetic client who has a community health nurse visit to:
   a. Draw up and administer 50 units of NPH insulin
   b. Provide foot care and review the 2000-calorie American Diabetes Association (ADA) diet
   c. Bring a supply of syringes and glucometer strips
   d. Observe insulin administration and foot care technique

9. Rogers' theory of the Science of Unitary Human Beings is best demonstrated by a community health nurse who:
   a. Encourages a client's interest in holistic health and therapeutic touch
   b. Focuses on the client's ability to cope successfully with family stress

c. Promotes the client's independence in meeting health care needs

d. Approaches the client knowing he is part of larger systems with which he interacts

10. An example of a class conducted by a community health nurse who uses the Knowles Adult Learning Theory would include:

a. Objectives written by the nurse in advance of the class to save the adults time

b. Structuring the class in a manner that gets the most information covered

c. Experiences built on the student's experiences and self-evaluation

d. Continuous teacher evaluations so the student knows if he or she is succeeding

ANSWER KEY

1. *Correct response: b*
Answer choices **a, c,** and **d** do not correctly define a theory. Ideas are associated, ideas are based on experience that is supported by data, and theories describe but do not change a phenomenon.
Comprehension/NA/NA

2. *Correct response: c*
Answer choices **a, b,** and **d** do not correctly describe why nursing theories are used. Nursing theories are not designed to control a client's life. They do not help nurses organize their day, nor do they provide a way to conduct practice. They may guide a nurse's view of practice through the description or explanation of nursing.
Application/NA/NA

3. *Correct response: a*
Answer choices **b, c,** and **d** do not depict the value of a nursing theory to community health nursing practice. Poverty, health care access, and destruction of the environment are elements of community health nursing practice but not as suggested in the remaining answer choices.
Comprehension/NA/NA

4. *Correct response: c*
Answer choices **a, b,** and **d** do not describe community health nursing. Care focuses on the primary level of prevention. Public health and basic nursing are blended, but all of the concepts not the "best." Care is directed toward all people; however, those who need and use the services most often have the least resources.
Application/Health Promotion/Analysis

5. *Correct response: d*
Answer choices **a, b,** and **c,** are theorists associated with the Science of Unitary Human Beings, Self-Care Theory and Adult Learning Theory, respectively.
Knowledge/NA/NA

6. *Correct response: a*
Answer choices **b, c,** and **d** do not describe an open system. Because a system is open and exchanges matter, energy, and information with its environment, stability and adaptiveness occur interchangeably as needed. If change is rapid, there may be temporary chaos or functional disruption. Matter on earth and in the universe is abundant and is constantly interacting.
Comprehension/NA/Assessment

7. *Correct response: c*
Answer choices **a, b,** and **d** do not describe clients who are adapting in a healthy manner.
Analysis/Psychosocial/Implementation

8. *Correct response: d*
Answer choices **a, b,** and **c** do not demonstrate the constructs of the self-care theory as well as answer choice **d.** In each incorrect response, the nurse is doing an activity that the client should be encouraged, taught, and observed doing him- or herself or they are activities a family member, caregiver, or neighbor could be taught to do for the client.
*Analysis/Health Promotion/
Implementation*

9. *Correct response: a*
Answer choices **b, c,** and **d** describe activities a nurse may focus on if following the nursing theories of Roy, Orem, and Neuman.
*Analysis/Health Promotion/
Implementation*

10. *Correct response: c*
Answer choices **a, b,** and **d** do not describe the use of adult learning theory. In adult learning theory, objectives would be written with the students, class structure would reflect the student's needs, and the teacher may give continuous feedback but not evaluation.
Analysis/Safe Care/Evaluation

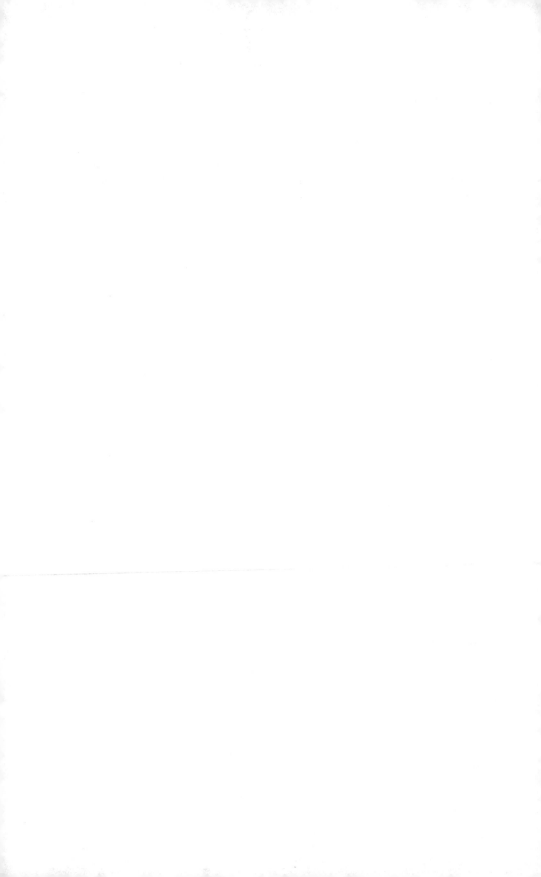

The Nursing Process Applied to Various Community Settings

I. Day Care Centers
A. Centers for Children

1. Services are provided for the child from birth to after-school care.

2. Services are offered in private homes or freestanding centers. They are also offered in secondary school, retirement or skilled nursing centers.

3. A license is required in most states when providing care for six or more children.

        4.   The fee varies depending on family income, program quality, and any additional services provided (extended hours, transportation, special lessons or trips).

        5.   Informal services focus on personal caregiving of the infant or child's basic needs. Formal services, on the other hand, focus on age-appropriate education, modeled after the ideas of educational theorists, such as Piaget or Montessori.

        6.   The qualifications of the caregiver range from none to specialized educational degrees.

B.   Centers for the Older Adult

        1.   In most communities, day care centers exist for lonely, frail, or adults with various forms of dementia.

        2.   Services are offered in homes or freestanding centers. They may also be associated with hospitals or skilled nursing facilities.

        3.   A license is required in most states.

        4.   The fees are generally moderate.

        5.   The service enables adult child caregivers to continue to work or have a respite from caregiving.

        6.   The services can be basic (food, shelter, safety) or comprehensive (doctor's appointments, therapies, trips, and entertainment).

        7.   The qualifications of the caregiver range from none to advanced medical, nursing, or educational degrees.

C.   The Nursing Process

        1.   Assessment: of needs to meet licensing requirements; to meet the present and future needs of the attendees

        2.   Nursing diagnoses
            a.   Anxiety
            b.   Compromised Family Coping
            c.   High Risk for Injury
            d.   Impaired Adjustment
            e.   Impaired Verbal Communication
            f.   Knowledge Deficit
            g.   Self-care Deficit
            h.   Sensory-Perceptual Alterations

        3.   Planning: work with administration and staff of day care centers to meet established goals and bring about needed and desired outcomes

        4.   Implementation
            a.   Monitoring to meet state regulations
            b.   Monitoring and/or administering immunizations
            c.   Observing for and monitoring infection control, safety, safe medication administration, toileting facilities, and food preparation and storage

      d. Educating staff on health and safety principles

      e. Educating attendees on health and safety practices

      f. Working collaboratively with interdisciplinary team members including administration and community leaders

      g. Being available for consultation on health and safety issues

  5. Evaluation: health and safety codes are met; health education needs of staff and participants are ongoing; consultative role has been established and is ongoing; issues presented in nursing diagnosis have been resolved

II. Schools

A. Preschools

  1. Private

      a. Age limit requirements (usually age 2 to 5)

      b. Child must have bowel and bladder control for most programs

      c. May have a small number of "scholarships" or parent aide programs to decrease cost and increase parental involvement

      d. Services as above—day care centers

  2. Head Start Programs

      a. Age 3 to 5

      b. Preparation for public school

      c. Federally funded comprehensive early childhood program for low-income children

      d. Not all eligible children are being reached

B. Public and Private Schools

  1. Elementary

      a. Children receive a formal education from kindergarten through eighth grade.

      b. Attendance is required of all children in every state, regardless of intellectual or physical ability, income, or place of residence.

      c. Special services are provided for developmentally delayed and physically challenged students.

      d. Public: Attendance is free, supported by public taxes; Private: Fees vary, can be very expensive.

      e. Transportation is provided for children living certain distances from school.

      f. Limited extracurricular activities are available to enrich the student experience.

  2. Secondary

      a. Children receive a formal education from ninth through twelfth grade.

   b. Attendance is required through age 16 in most states. It is, however, difficult to monitor, and many students fail to graduate.

   c. Accessibility is the same as in elementary school.

   d. Extracurricular activities are available to enrich the student experience (in some schools with unlimited resources, the extracurricular activities are abundant).

  3. Home school

   a. An option in most states for families who so choose to educate their children at home

   b. Curricular materials available from and monitored by the state

   c. Extracurricular activities generally not part of home school programs

C. **Colleges and Universities**

 1. Higher education is not a required part of the educational process in the United States.

 2. Colleges and universities are supported by private or public funds.

 3. Educational experiences vary in relation to campus size, location, financial support, courses offered, auxiliary services, and institutional mission.

D. **Commonalities Among all Schools**

 1. The goal of all formal educational programs is to have a child in the healthiest state possible, in the healthiest environment possible, so learning can take place.

 2. Most educational institutions have access to health care services and the services of a community health nurse (CHN).

 3. Some school districts hire school nurses to serve their schools. Nurses become part of the educational program and provide a wide variety of services for the students, faculty, and staff. The district expense is similar to the cost of a teacher.

 4. Other school districts contract for the services of a CHN through the local public health department. The services provided are not as extensive due to other responsibilities in the public health department. Services are less expensive for the school district.

 5. Services in elementary, secondary, and higher educational settings are similar and are adjusted to meet the needs of the developmental age of the population.

 6. The nurse's role is extensive and includes monitoring, screening, providing care, counseling, teaching (Display 10-1).

E. **The Nursing Process**

 1. Assessment: of needs to meet state requirements; to meet the educational goals of the school district or college; to meet the present and future needs of the students

DISPLAY 10-1.
The Expanded Role of the School (Campus) Nurse

> ► Monitor the health and safety of the facility
> ► Monitor health records
>   (new and existing students)
> ► Provide selected screening or health care services
>   (vision, hearing, scoliosis, physical examinations)
> ► Assist with first-aid
> ► Teach students, faculty, and staff
>   (formally and informally)
> ► Collaborate with faculty on health curriculum
> ► Serve on school and community health-related committees
> ► Make home visits to high-risk families
> ► Provide selected immunizations to students and staff
> ► Provide health and personal counseling
>   (within the job description)
> ► Make appropriate referrals and follow up on them
> ► Work collaboratively with other personnel for the benefit
>   of the student
> ► Sponsor or assist with health fairs, health careers clubs
> ► Participate in other health-related activities unique to the
>   school setting

2. Nursing diagnoses:
   a. Altered Role Performance
   b. Decisional Conflict
   c. High Risk for Injury
   d. Impaired Adjustment
   e. Knowledge Deficit
3. Planning: work with administration and staff in the educational institution to meet established goals and bring about needed and desired outcomes
4. Implementation
   a. Monitoring to meet state regulations
   b. Monitoring and/or administering immunizations and other medications within the scope of practice and philosophy of the educational institution
   c. Observing for and monitoring infection control, safety, safe medication administration, toileting facilities, and food preparation and storage
   d. Educating staff on health and safety principles
   e. Educating students on health and safety practices
   f. Working collaboratively with interdisciplinary team members including administration and community leaders
   g. Being available for consultation on health and safety issues
   h. Serving on campus-wide health-related committees
5. Evaluation: health and safety codes are met; health education needs of staff and students are ongoing; consultative role has

been established and is ongoing; issues presented in nursing diagnoses have been resolved

III.   Work Settings

A.   Offices

1.   Setting description: indoor work; 5 days a week; sedentary, repetitive activities; commuting (an average of 11 miles each way for each employee in the United States)
2.   Employee description: all ages, races, and genders; all levels of skill and education
3.   Ergonomic factors (the design of workplaces, tools, and tasks that are compatible with the person): the lighting; temperature; extended periods of sitting, hours of computer use; repetitive activities; stress of deadlines

B.   Industries

1.   Setting description: predominantly indoor work; temperatures may vary with the type of manufacturing process; physical labor expected, often extreme; assembly line jobs are repetitive; number of coworkers larger than in offices
2.   Employee description: all ages, races, and genders (tends to be more male and minority); skill and education vary (tend to be more highly skilled with less formal education); owners and managers predominantly white males; foremen and supervisors a more equal racial mix but remains male dominated
3.   Ergonomic factors: lighting; heat; noise; lifting; standing for long periods; odors; exposure to toxic substances; boredom

C.   Agricultural Settings

1.   Setting description (in the United States): most agricultural operations are large, employing unrelated seasonal workers; small family-owned and -operated farms are declining in number; setting is outdoors, predominantly in warm or hot weather; health care and retirement benefits not usually provided
2.   Employee description
    a.   Owner and family members: motivation to work based on family loyalties and success of own business venture
    b.   Legal migrant workers: may be hired seasonally or by the day; wages based on season, skill and supply of work and employees; workers are of all ages, races; tend to be low to low-middle income, nonwhite male workers or families; housing is often provided but is substandard to abusive
    c.   Illegal migrant workers: there is a growing number of illegal immigrants from Mexico who work for low wages in agriculture; the wages are low but are much higher than similar work in Mexico
3.   Ergonomic factors: outdoor work; extreme temperatures; long workdays; physically laborious with heavy lifting and bending;

inhalation of pesticides, skin exposure to poisons, sun exposure; limited access to toileting facilities; seasonal work

D. The Nursing Process

1. Assessment: of needs to meet federal, state, and local health and safety requirements; to meet the employment goals of the work setting; to meet the present and future needs of the employees

2. Nursing diagnoses
   a. Altered Role Performance
   b. Decisional Conflict
   c. High Risk for Injury
   d. Knowledge Deficit

3. Planning: work with administration, staff, and employee groups in work settings to meet established goals and bring about needed and desired outcomes

4. Implementation
   a. Monitoring to meet federal, state, and local regulations
   b. Delivering a variety of health care services deemed necessary to ensure employee health and safety within the scope of practice and philosophy of the work setting
   c. Observing for meeting OSHA regulations in and around the work setting (in private industry and the federal sector)
   d. Educating administration and management on health and safety principles
   e. Educating employees on health and safety practices
   f. Being available for consultation on health and safety issues
   g. Working collaboratively with interdisciplinary team members including administration and management
   h. Serving on industry-wide health-related committees

5. Evaluation: health and safety codes are met; health education needs of staff and employees are ongoing; consultative role has been established and is ongoing; issues presented in nursing diagnoses have been resolved

IV. Outpatient Settings

A. Public and Private Clinics

1. These services are offered for all ages and focus on medical, surgical, and preventive needs.

2. Both private and public clinics provide comprehensive services.

3. The differences between private and public clinics include funding sources; client's payment source; educational preparation and experience of staff; services provided.

B. **Same-Day Surgical Centers**

1. Provides surgical interventions on an outpatient basis; is an extended service of an existing public or private acute care health facility or it is a freestanding center, privately owned; avoids an overnight stay in a facility for clients in stable health condition needing elective surgery of a minor to minimal risk situation for more major interventions

2. Procedures include appendectomy, hernia repair, tubal ligation, vasectomy, tonsillectomy, cataract and other eye surgeries, cosmetic and reconstructive surgery

 3. **Purpose: cost savings; clients recover at home; infection reduction rate**

4. CHNs may work in the clinic or same-day surgical setting (role is similar to acute care nursing (refer to Lippincott Review Series: *Medical-Surgical Nursing*, 1996); CHNs may make follow-up visits to clients at home between clinic visits. (See Section V, this chapter.) CHNs provide follow-up postsurgical intervention at home after same-day surgery (see role of the home health nurse, Section V, Chapter 18)

V. **Homes: The purpose of home visits is to provide traditional community health nursing services (Chap. 5, Section II:C) and home health and hospice nursing services (see Chap. 20).**

A. Private Dwellings—residences inhabited by one family; consisting of one or more members; may be a house or an apartment with inhabitants

B. **Congregate Living Settings**

1. Larger homelike settings resembling apartment buildings
2. Designed for semi-independent and assisted living
3. Individual "apartments" are small (studio to one or two bedrooms)
4. May have very limited cooking facilities
5. Dining room service is provided for most meals
6. Housekeeping and laundry services provided
7. Minimal assistance with care may be provided
8. Residents are aged or disabled
9. Occupancy may be in the hundreds
10. Licensed by the state
11. Staff more inclusive: dietary personnel, activity therapists, resident managers, and minimal nursing staff

C. Residential Care Facilities: established for residents who need a higher level of caregiving due to age or disability; provided in a family's own home or in a homelike setting established specifically for board and care purposes; licensed by the state; usually serving four or more residents; staff at the nursing assistant level, numbers based on occupancy and resident dependency

D. Skilled Nursing Facilities

    1.   Clients needing more skilled care become residents of skilled nursing facilities, inpatient hospices, or acute care hospitals.

    2.   CHNs do not routinely make visits in these settings because they are staffed with appropriate health care practitioners, except when consulting or discharge planning to promote continuity of care.

E. The Nursing Process

    1.   Assessment: of needs to meet federal, state, and local health and safety requirements; to meet individual client present and future needs

    2.   Nursing diagnoses (may encompass the entire range of established nursing diagnoses)

        a.   Altered Health Maintenance

        b.   Altered Nutrition

        c.   Altered Role Performance

        d.   Decisional Conflict

        e.   High Risk for Injury

        f.   Impaired Physical Mobility

        g.   Impaired Social Interaction

        h.   Ineffective Management of Therapeutic Regimen

        i.   Knowledge Deficit

        j.   Self-esteem Disturbance

        k.   Social Isolation

    3.   Planning: work with administration, staff, resident, and resident groups to meet established goals and bring about needed and desired outcomes in the individual or setting

    4.   Implementation

        a.   Monitoring to meet federal, state, and local regulations

        b.   Delivering a variety of health care services deemed necessary to ensure resident health and safety within the scope of practice and philosophy of the residence

        c.   Educating administration and management on health and safety principles

        d.   Educating residents on health and safety practices

        e.   Being available for consultation on health and safety issues

        f.   Working collaboratively with interdisciplinary team members including administration and management

        g.   Serving on health-related committees

    5.   Evaluation: health and safety codes are met; health education needs of staff and employees are ongoing; consultative role has been established and is ongoing; issues presented in nursing diagnosis have been resolved

VI. Incarceration Facilities

A. Prisons

1. Nationwide system of facilities designed to secure those awaiting trial for an offense or those serving a sentence for an offense
2. Millions of people nationwide are incarcerated. 1995 was the first year the California state budget for the incarcerated exceeded the state budget for higher education.
3. This is a growing population with increasingly complex health and social needs.
4. Facilities are at the local, state, and federal level.
5. Physical design is based on the security needs of the inmates, ranging from isolation, high security, trustee programs, and work release programs.
6. The population is increasingly young and minority, with an average age of 21 and a disproportionate racial mix of African Americans and Latino Americans.

B. Prison Hospitals

1. Some facilities separate mentally ill criminals from the main population.
2. Health care needs are great; diseases and conditions have the potential to occur in epidemic proportions, such as HIV/AIDS, tuberculosis, skin infections, dental caries, accidents, personal injury from violence against one another, substance abuse.

C. The Nursing Process

1. Assessment: of needs to meet licensing requirements; to meet the present and future needs of the incarcerated
2. Nursing diagnoses
   a. Altered Health Maintenance
   b. Altered Protection
   c. Altered Role Performance
   d. Decisional Conflict
   e. High Risk for Caregiver Role Strain
   f. High Risk for Injury
   g. High Risk for Self-mutilation
   h. High Risk for Trauma
   i. High Risk for Violence, directed at self/others
   j. Impaired Social Interaction
   k. Knowledge Deficit
   l. Social Isolation
3. Planning: work with administration and security staff of the facility to meet established goals of this secure environment, and bring about needed and desired health- and safety-related outcomes

4. Implementation
   a. Monitoring to meet federal and state regulations
   b. Administering a health and wellness program focusing on primary prevention
   c. Observing for and monitoring infection control, safety and security, safe medication administration
   d. Educating staff and the incarcerated on health and safety principles and practices
   e. Working collaboratively with interdisciplinary team members including administration, staff, and community leaders
   f. Being available for consultation on health and safety issues
5. Evaluation: health and safety codes are met; health education needs of staff and the incarcerated are ongoing; consultative role has been established and is ongoing; issues presented in nursing diagnoses have been successfully resolved

VII. Other Settings
A. Homeless Shelters
1. Shelters provide: minimal services of overnight shelter to a select few persons; comprehensive family-focused services including three meals a day, health care services, and social, educational, and work training programs
2. The population is of all ages from all walks of life; single, married, and families
3. CHN role: may resemble "curbside" nursing (see C. below) or be as comprehensive as a multiservice clinic (see section IV, this chapter)

B. Senior and Youth Centers
1. Centers provide recreational services and meals for members; minimal screening and health promotion services; comprehensive in nature with fully staffed medical, social, and recreational programs.
2. Membership in centers occurs in all communities; rural, suburban, inner city, members are from all social, economic, and wellness levels.
3. CHN role: minimal and voluntary; similar to outpatient CHN services; comprehensive and innovative in nature

C. "Storefront" and "Curbside" Settings
1. Nurses provide impromptu and innovative services based on observed needs that are urgent in nature, occur in particular situations, and are met in no other way.
2. The population varies and includes homeless, alcohol-dependent persons, tuberculosis clients, substance abusers, teen runaways.

3.   CHN role: depends on the nature of the client needs; commitment of the nurse to initiate services; procurement of needed resources through interdisciplinary collaboration

Bibliography

Brown, M. L. (1988). An historical perspective: One hundred years of industrial or occupational health nursing in the United States. *AAOHN Journal, 41*(1), 8–15.

Eliopoulos, C. (1993). *Gerontological nursing* (3rd ed.). Philadelphia: J.B. Lippincott.

Lindsey, A. M. (1989). Health care for the homeless. *Nursing Outlook, 37*(2), 78.

Spradley, B. W., & Allender, J. A. (1996). *Community health nursing: Concepts and practice.* (4th ed.). Philadelphia: Lippincott-Raven.

Zanga, J. R., & Oda, D. S. (1987). School health services. *Journal of School Health, 57*(10), 413–416.

STUDY QUESTIONS

1. The role of the CHN when working with child and adult day care centers includes:
   a. Managing the day-to-day operation of the center
   b. Fund raising to procure needed equipment and supplies
   c. Working with administration to assess the needs of the attendees
   d. Developing goals that meet international guidelines for caregiving

2. The role of the CHN in the public school system includes:
   a. The same responsibilities and activities as the teachers
   b. A broad base of services to provide a healthy school environment
   c. Discipline and exclusion of children breaking school rules
   d. Planning and implementing the health curriculum

3. A CHN in a work setting spends the day conducting employee physicals, assessing the worksite for safety hazards, and conducting a first aid course for middle managers. This nurse most likely works for:
   a. A large insurance company
   b. A farming conglomerate
   c. A chain of department stores
   d. An automobile assembly plant

4. Ergonomic factors in the work setting include the:
   a. Design, tools, and tasks of the workplace
   b. Financial stability of the organization
   c. Ethnic and racial mix of employees
   d. Speed with which the company grows

5. Special health and safety concerns of the agricultural work setting include:
   a. Boredom, repetitious activities, and noise pollution
   b. Exposure to toxic substances and weather extremes

   c. Emotional stress of meeting deadlines and conflict of interests
   d. Sitting for long hours with prolonged periods of inactivity

6. The main purpose for having a CHN in schools or at the work site is to:
   a. Provide primary prevention services to a generally healthy population
   b. Be available to administer first-aid when needed by students or employees
   c. Be sure the school or company is meeting federal and state regulations
   d. Attend to the needs of the physically and emotionally disabled

7. A congregate living setting can be identified by the following characteristics:
   a. A building made of concrete with limited use of wood or wood products
   b. Small private living quarters with group dining and some social services
   c. A private residence inhabited by one family with one or more members
   d. Residents who are highly dependent with skilled nursing needs

8. When working with the incarcerated, there is *one* major difference from other settings that CHNs work in:
   a. The clients may be physically abusive.
   b. The population is generally healthy.
   c. Safety and security are the first responsibility.
   d. The clients do not want health care services.

9. Providing community health nursing services to aggregates in the community has many positive benefits including the cost-effective nature of:
   a. Primary prevention
   b. Secondary prevention

    c. Tertiary prevention

    d. Diagnostic Related Groupings (DRGs)

10. CHN services have an influence on the health of individuals as demonstrated by:

    a. An increase in clients using the acute care setting for hospital admission

    b. Hospitalized clients being more knowledgeable about their health

    c. Clients having the skills necessary to maintain a higher level of wellness

    d. Clients caring for themselves and not using any health care services

ANSWER KEY

1. *Correct response: c*

Answer choices **a** and **b** are roles of the administration and staff.

Answer choice **d:** there are no international guidelines for caregiving.

Application/NA/Implementation

2. *Correct response: b*

Answer choices **a, c,** and **d** describe roles of teachers and administrators.

Application/Safe Care/Implementation

3. *Correct response: d*

Answer choices **a** and **c** describe businesses without foremen or significant safety hazards the nurse would be able to assess within the work day, especially in a chain of department stores.

Answer choice **b** is agricultural, and the activities described are not a practical part of a nurse's role when working in an agricultural setting.

Application/Safe Care/Implementation

4. *Correct response: a*

Answer choices **b, c,** and **d** are not related to the ergonomic factors of the work setting.

Application/Safe Care/Implementation

5. *Correct response: b*

Answer choice **a** describes an agricultural setting.

Answer choices **c** and **d** better describe the business setting.

Analysis/Safe Care/Implementation

6. *Correct response: a*

Answer choices **b, c,** and **d** may be activities of the nurse in the described settings but are not the main purpose for having a nurse in the setting.

Analysis/NA/Evaluation

7. *Correct response: b*

Answer choice **a** describes the physical characteristics of a certain type of structure.

Answer choice **c** describes a private home.

Answer choice **d** describes a skilled nursing facility.

Application/NA/Analysis

8. *Correct response: c*

Answer choices **a, b,** and **d** may apply to any setting. In prisons and jails, the purpose of the facility is security. Health needs, no matter how severe, are secondary.

Application/Safe Care/Analysis

9. *Correct response: a*

Primary care is the most cost-effective. Secondary is more expensive. Tertiary care is the most expensive. DRGs may reduce costs in acute care settings but do not directly affect costs in the community.

Comprehension/NA/Analysis

10. *Correct response: c*

Answer choice **a, b,** and **d** are not the goals of community health nursing. However, if clients need inpatient care, it is desirable that they be more knowledgeable about their health and health care. They should be able to provide effective self-care, but when health services are needed the client should know when and how to access it.

Analysis/Safe Care/Evaluation

Research in Community Health Nursing

I. Research

A. Purpose

1. **Expand the scope of practice**
2. Strengthen nursing theory
3. Improve care given to clients
4. Improve the health of clients

B. Participation

1. Collaborate in the development of an idea for a research project
2. Participate actively in the implementation of scientific studies in the work setting
3. Prepare academically for the leadership role in conducting research; acquire appropriate tools and resources to enhance grant writing skills to fund research; understand and use the research process and statistics

C. Examples
1. Maternal and child health
2. Tuberculosis
3. Health response as people seek to restore or promote health
4. Cost of specific health care interventions
5. Measurement of levels of wellness

D. Organizations and Journals
1. National Institute of Nursing Research—full institute status within the National Institutes of Health in 1993
    a. Purpose: to promote and financially support research training and research relating to client care
    b. Services: research reference materials, education, consultation, funding
    c. Institute agenda
        1995—community-based nursing models
        1996—effectiveness of nursing intervention in HIV/AIDS
        1997—cognitive impairment
        1998—living with chronic illness
        1999—biobehavioral factors related to improve immunocompetence
2. American Nurses Association Center for Research in Nursing—established in 1983
    a. Purpose: to develop and coordinate a research program to serve as the source of national data for the profession
    b. Priority: to help focus research more precisely on aspects of nursing practice
3. Sigma Theta Tau—The International Nursing Honor Society
    a. Purpose: to recognize and promote excellence in nursing
    b. Services: funding of nursing research, research conferences (international, national, and those sponsored by local chapters), a nursing journal, online journal services, Virginia Henderson research library
4. Major Nursing Research Journals
    a. *Nursing Research*
    b. *Advances in Nursing Science*
    c. *Western Journal of Nursing Research*
    d. *Applied Nursing Research*
    e. *Clinical Nursing Research*
    f. *Qualitative Health Research*
    g. *Image*
    h. *Journal of Public Health Nursing*
    i. *American Journal of Public Health* (not just nursing research)

II.   Research Approaches
A.   Quantitative
1.   Definition
   a.   Collection of data on things that can be quantified or measured objectively
   b.   Studies tend to focus on parts of, rather than the whole of, an experience or phenomenon
2.   Methods
   a.   Self-reports: questionnaires, telephone surveys
   b.   Observation: a record of behaviors or events
   c.   Biophysiologic measures: measurement of physiologic functions
3.   Examples
   a.   Compare data between two ways of doing things, such as cloth vs disposable diapers for contamination or cost
   b.   Quantify the knowledge level of people on health-related subjects, such as how to prevent HIV/AIDS or to do breast self-examination
   c.   Assess the client's use of health-related behaviors, such as safe sex practices or breast self-examinations
   d.   Determine a child's hemoglobin, blood lead level, or the blood sugar of a diabetic after initiating dietary or safety changes

B.   Qualitative
1.   Definition
   a.   Emphasize subjectivity or the meaning of experiences for individuals
   b.   More holistic in nature than quantitative studies; attempt to understand a problem or phenomenon
2.   Methods
   a.   Case studies
   b.   Ethnography
   c.   Historical research
   d.   Observation, field studies
   e.   Phenomenology
3.   Examples
   a.   Initiate a survey of homeless people to determine what they perceive as barriers to receiving health care
   b.   Conduct interviews with school nurses to determine what they perceive as their role in the school and community
   c.   Observe participants of an adult day care center to document their use of time, initiative in activities, and interaction with one another

III.   The Research Process
A.   Assessment
1.   Identify an area of interest
   a.   Select an observed phenomenon from the clinical setting
   b.   Explore questions you have about clients; caregiver role; agency services; broader health issues
2.   Begin an initial review of the literature
   a.   Conduct a broad survey of the topic
   b.   Provides investigator direction and focus
3.   Identify the population

B.   Planning

1.   **Formulate a research question (determine the questions in need of answers)**
   a.   Research questions: questions in need of answers (What is the frequency of mothers under the age of 20 following through with immunizations on their children under the age of 2? What are the barriers to receiving health care for young mothers who are under the age of 20?)
   b.   Hypotheses: statements made about a phenomenon from a specific directional approach (Young mothers under the age of 20 do not follow through with immunizations for their children under the age of 2 as frequently as mothers who are over the age of 20. As a null hypothesis, the statement would be worded: There is no difference between the mother's age and immunization frequency.)
2.   Select a conceptual model
   a.   Provides a way of organizing phenomena
   b.   Serves as the preliminary steps in the construction of more formal theories
   c.   Develops future research
3.   Choose a research design
   a.   Serves as the overall plan for how to obtain answers to the questions being studied
   b.   Includes a wide variety of experimental or nonexperimental designs
   c.   Guides three types of studies:

   ▶ Retrospective: conducted from existing data (reviewing clinic charts from the past year on the hemoglobin levels of children under the age of 5)
   ▶ Prospective: conducted from current data (asking clients receiving home visits during a 1-month period to answer questions about their current tobacco use)
   ▶ Longitudinal studies: conducted over long periods of time (following infants born in one town during a 6-month period through age 8 to monitor height and weight information correlated with birth weight, birth order, and number of siblings)

C. Implementation

    1. Select sample participants

        a. Select samples of the intended population because it is not practical to reach all people

          ▶ Random selection: all population members have an equal chance of being selected

          ▶ Convenience sample: population members, meeting the criteria, are selected because they can be reached and agree to participate (women using one clinic or the fifth grade classroom in a neighborhood school)

        b. Human subject rights: inform participants of their risks and right to withdraw from the study whenever they want; ensure confidentiality, obtain parental permission if participant is a minor

    2. Collect data

        a. Train multiple data collectors to follow protocol in order to protect the integrity of the study

        b. Protect the human subject rights for all participants

        c. Keep precise records of collected data in a form ready for analysis

D. Evaluation

    1. Analyze findings

        a. Use a variety of appropriate statistical manipulations that assist with data analysis

        b. Select and use correct statistics (or have a statistician as a research team member)

        c. Compile results in a format to prepare for interpretation

    2. Interpret results

        a. Explain the results in a manner to be understood by intended audiences

        b. Answer each research question or explain each hypothesis and whether it is supported or not supported

E. Action

    1. **Communicate findings**

        a. Write up results and submit to an appropriate nursing research journal or other professional publication

        b. Present findings to colleagues at all levels through international, national, regional, state, or local research conferences

    2. Apply results to improve a nursing practice or improve the health of clients

IV. **Research Funding**

    A. **Federal Grants: joint funding between several federal agencies or organizations; monies can be into the millions**

        1. US Public Health Service

      2. Department of Health and Human Services

      3. American Public Health Association

      4. American Red Cross

      5. American Cancer Society

B. **State Grants: joint funding between interested agencies at the state level; monies can be into the hundreds of thousands**

      1. State health departments

      2. State automobile associations

      3. State nurses' association

C. **Organizational Grants: offered by specific organizations, companies, institutes, or foundations; amounts vary**

      1. Health maintenance organizations

      2. National or regional companies

D. **Local or Regional Grants: health care systems, special interest groups, individuals; amounts vary**

      1. Local companies

      2. Local charities

E. **Researcher Grants**

      1. Select funding source applications from groups that match extent of the proposed project, direction of the research, group the research will benefit

      2. Acquire needed application forms; complete in detail; submit by the deadline

      3. If funding is granted; maintain deadlines, conduct study as presented on the application, keep funding source informed as requested; stay within budget

      4. If funding is not granted; submit to another funding source or rewrite and resubmit

      5. Present findings as required by the funding source in addition to other methods deemed appropriate

      6. Use information from initial research to develop new research projects

V. **The Role of the Community Health Nurse in Research**

    A. **Participate in Research-Related Activities**

      1. Participate in a journal club in the practice setting where regular meetings among community health nurses occur to discuss and critique research articles

      2. Attend national research presentations at professional conferences such as the Annual Meeting of the American Public Health Association (APHA); local research conferences sponsored by schools of nursing or health departments

      3. Join the International Nursing Honor Society—Sigma Theta Tau; read the research in their journal, *Image*; use their online journal and research library services

    4. Subscribe to practice setting appropriate and generic research journals, such as *Journal of Public Health Nursing* and *Nursing Research*

B. Collaborate on Research Projects

    1. Use of expertise
       a. Accessibility to and knowledge of subjects
       b. Data gathering
       c. Assist with data analysis
       d. Co-present or assist with writing the results to disseminate findings in professional publications

    2. Interprofessional role: research projects involve various professionals such as physicians, social workers, health educators, and psychologists
       a. Provide accessibility to subjects
       b. Share clinical expertise regarding the subjects
       c. Gather nursing data
       d. Assist with data analysis
       e. Co-present or assist with writing the results with interprofessional members to disseminate findings to groups and in journals from a variety of professions

C. Apply Research Findings in the Community

    1. Use information found in nursing research articles to benefit clients served
    2. Participate on an organizational committee whose mission is to review the ethical aspects of proposed research involving clients, before it is undertaken (help to establish such a group if one does not exist in your agency)

D. Initiate Research Projects

    1. Access a funding source
       a. Determine purpose and extent of the study as a guide to potential funding sources
       b. Apply for funding in a timely manner

    2. Lead the research
       a. Guide the direction of the study and ensure the quality of the study
       b. Select and prepare co-investigators and research assistants
       c. Provide the funding source with periodic reports
       d. Meet the expectations of the study through to dissemination of results

Bibliography

Polit, D. F., & Hungler, B. P. (1995). *Nursing research: Principles and methods.* Philadelphia: J.B. Lippincott.

Smith, C. M., & Maurer, F. A. (1995). *Community health nursing: Theory and practice.* Philadelphia: W.B. Saunders.

Spradley, B. W., & Allender, J. A. (1996). *Community health nursing: Concepts and practice.* (4th ed.). Philadelphia: Lippincott-Raven.

Stanhope, M., & Lancaster, J. (1992). *Community health nursing: Process and practice for promoting health.* (3rd ed.). St. Louis: Mosby–Year Book.

STUDY QUESTIONS

1. Participation in nursing research by community health nurses requires:
   a. Application of nursing research to promote practice and client health status
   b. Advanced academic degrees with a focus on nursing research
   c. Ability to understand the various statistical manipulations used
   d. Collaboration with other professionals in the health care arena

2. Sigma Theta Tau, the International Nursing Honor Society, has as its purpose to:
   a. Serve as the source of national data for the profession
   b. Recognize and promote excellence in nursing
   c. Establish a yearly agenda of topics as a nursing research focus
   d. Help focus research more precisely on aspects of nursing practice

3. Several nursing journals have a research focus. One in particular is:
   a. *The American Journal of Nursing*
   b. *Nursing Outlook*
   c. *Nursing Times*
   d. *Advance in Nursing Science*

4. Which of the following research studies represents quantitative research?
   a. Comparing the weights of children with their hemoglobin levels
   b. Assessing what men perceive as their greatest health care issues
   c. Analyzing a group of children's bedtime routines and patterns
   d. Observing the infant bathing practices of new mothers

5. Which of the following research studies represents qualitative research?
   a. Comparing the weights of infants with amount and brand of formula taken
   b. Assessing the number of and reason for health care provider visits by men

   c. Analyzing a group of children's bedtime routines and patterns
   d. Observing women with toddlers in stores for the number of verbal reprimands

6. In the assessment phase of the research process, the researcher:
   a. Determines the questions in need of answers
   b. Selects a conceptual model to organize phenomena
   c. Chooses a research design that serves as an overall plan for the study
   d. Explores questions about clients, caregivers, and the health care system

7. In the implementation phase of the research process, the researcher:
   a. Selects a sample population to participate in the study
   b. Chooses a conceptual model to organize phenomena
   c. Chooses a research design that serves as an overall plan for the study
   d. Explores questions about clients, caregivers, and the health care system

8. In the action phase of the research process, the researcher:
   a. Selects a sample population to participate in the study
   b. Communicates findings in write-ups or presentations for professionals
   c. Chooses a research design that serves as an overall plan for the study
   d. Analyzes the findings and compiles them to prepare for interpretation

9. Which one of the following gives an example of a retrospective research study?
   a. A CHN interviewing older adults coming into a flu shot clinic this fall
   b. CHNs having families complete a questionnaire on home visits
   c. A clinic CHN reviewing charts of visits made by 2- and 3-year-old children last March

d. Several CHNs provide a service different from the rest of the agency nurses

10. As a consumer of nursing research, the community health nurse:
    a. Attends the national Sigma Theta Tau research conference
    b. Participates in research conducted in the local community
    c. Finds funding sources for research to be conducted in the future
    d. Leads a research study with interdisciplinary team members

ANSWER KEY

1. **Correct response: a**
   Answer choice **b.** An advanced degree is beneficial but not necessary to participate in nursing research.
   Answer choice **c.** The statistics used can be the domain of the principal investigator or a statistician.
   Answer choice **d.** Nurses can work on studies without collaboration that includes other professionals.
   Application/NA/Implementation

2. **Correct response: b**
   Answer choices **a** and **d** are the mission and a priority of the American Nurses' Association Center for Research for Nursing.
   Answer choice **c** is an activity of the National Institute of Nursing Research.
   Comprehension/NA/Analysis

3. **Correct response: d**
   Answer choices **a, b,** and **c** are popular nursing journals for practice-related thoughts and ideas that are not necessarily research based or presented as research articles.
   Comprehension/Safe Care/Planning

4. **Correct response: a**
   Answer choices **b, c,** and **d** describe samples of qualitative research where the meaning of experiences to individuals are described and studies tend to be more holistic in an attempt to understand a problem or phenomenon.
   Application/NA/Implementation

5. **Correct response: c**
   Answer choices **a, b,** and **d** are examples of quantitative research. Participants self-report on issues in question, certain behaviors are captured via observation or there is measurement of physiologic function.
   Application/NA/Implementation

6. **Correct response: d**
   Answer choices **a, b,** and **c** are examples of the planning phase.
   Application/NA/Implementation

7. **Correct response: a**
   Answer choices **b** and **c** are examples of the planning phase.
   Answer choice **d** is an example of the assessment phase.
   Application/NA/Implementation

8. **Correct response: b**
   Answer choice **a** is an example of the implementation phase.
   Answer choice **c** is an example of planning phase.
   Answer choice **d** is an example of the evaluation phase.
   Application/NA/Implementation

9. **Correct response: c**
   Answer choices **a, b,** and **d** are examples of a prospective study (with choice d being experimental).
   Application/NA/Implementation

10. **Correct response: a**
    Answer choices **b, c,** and **d** are examples of activities a community health nurse engages in as a researcher. A consumer learns about research being done by attending conferences, reading nursing research journals, and applying it in the clinical setting.
    Application/NA/Implementation

Unit IV
Protecting and Promoting the Health of People Throughout the Life Span

Influence of Diversity on Community Health

I. The Meaning of Diversity to Community Health Nursing

A. Description: Diversity is variety

1. The patterns of living that people choose are based on:
   a. Educational and financial resources
   b. Values and beliefs
2. The differences among people originate from:
   a. Genetic makeup
   b. Collective experiences
3. Cultural plurality coexists within communities

B. Significance

1. The client
   a. Diversity is a known; a norm for the person
   b. What is perceived as different by others may be seen as normal to the client

       c.   Seeks care from health care workers who are from diverse backgrounds

       d.   Expects quality care from any caregiver

  2. The health care worker

       a.   Works with diverse populations in every setting

       b.   Acknowledges, accepts, and works with the diversity of clients to provide relevant care

       c.   Recognizes the perception of diversity as significant

II. Types of Diversity

A. Cultural

  1. Definitions (Spradley & Allender, 1996)

       a.   *Culture:* the beliefs, values, and behavior that are shared by members of a society and that provide a design or "map" for living

       b.   *Cultural diversity:* the variety of cultural patterns that co-exist within a designated geographic area

       c.   *Race:* a biologically designated group of people whose distinguishing features are inherited

       d.   *Ethnicity:* the qualities that mark one's association with an ethnic group

       e.   *Ethnic group:* a collection of people with common origins and with shared culture and identity

  2. United States

       a.   Over one hundred different ethnic groups live in the United States

m   b.   **There are three ethnic groups of significant size; Hispanic Americans, African Americans, Asian Americans (Display 12-1).**

       c.   Immigration patterns have changed over the decades. In

DISPLAY 12-1.
Projected Changes in Large Minority Groups in the U.S.

MINORITY GROUP	NUMBER	1990 % OF POP.	2050 ESTIMATED % OF POP.
African Americans	30 million	12%	15%
Hispanic Americans*	22 million	9%	21%
Asian Americans[†]	7 million	3%	10%
		24%	46%[‡]

*%in the population more than doubles in 60 years.
[†]% in the population more than triples in 60 years.
[‡]These three minority groups will make up almost half of the US population.

the 1800s and early 1900s, immigration was from northern and eastern European countries; however, since the 1960s, immigration has shifted to Asian and Latino countries.

B.   Gender and Age
    1. People of all ages live in the United States.
    2. The population in the United States is getting older.

    3. 85 years and older: the fastest growing segment of the population
    4. Specific gender and age differences
        a. A fairly equal number of males and females are born each year.
        b. Through age 25, more males die prematurely related to drownings, bicycle and automobile crashes; violence involving guns; AIDS.
        c. Age 25 to 40, men and women have fairly equal death rates.
        d. After age 40, more males die prematurely from cardiac and coronary artery diseases; cancers affect both sexes equally, although the sites of origin may differ.
        e. By age 80, females outnumber males two to one and the spread increases as elders age.

C.   Other Types
    1. Income and social status
        a. In a democracy, differences in income are great
        b. In the United States, people live in the poorest of conditions, resembling life in third-world countries, to the most extravagant lifestyles imaginable.
        c. The majority of citizens are of middle income, never experiencing the extravagant lifestyle.

        d. Social status in the United States is not predetermined by birth, as in some cultures, but is tied more closely to education and income.

        e. The services provided by public health agencies tend to be directed to people in poverty or of low income. The caregiving focuses on groups with a common factor of low income.
    2. Sexual orientation
        a. About 10% of people are homosexual (prefer sexual contact with people of their own gender).
        b. This is a recognized group possessing significant political power.
        c. It is fairly recent that acceptance of the gay lifestyle has occurred.

        d.   Because the gay lifestyle is not an acceptable alternative to some people, there is often conflicting messages given by the larger community regarding this lifestyle choice.

        e.   The disregard for the gay community may have delayed investigation into the cause and prevention of AIDS in the earliest years of the epidemic, thus affecting the health of all members of society.

   3.   Physical or mental

        a.   Many members of society suffer challenging physical and mental diversities that can be barriers to a quality life.

        b.   Some of the major preventable causes include: premature birth, alcohol use during pregnancy, substance abuse, victims of violence, automobile crashes, cerebral vascular accidents.

        c.   Through medical, technological and computer advances, along with client advocacy, the physically and mentally challenged successfully coexist in society, in schools, at play, and in the work setting.

III. Ethnocentrism

A.   **Definition:** *ethnocentrism* **is the belief and feeling that one's own culture is best and right where other groups are inferior or wrong**

B.   **Clients and the Practice Setting**

   1.   Health care workers who approach clients from an ethnocentric perspective are unable to give appropriate care.

   2.   Ethnocentrism may be conscious or unconscious and involves a lack of understanding or appreciation of other beliefs and practices.

   3.   Ethnocentric feelings affect practice, causing care to be nonexistent or, at best, marginal.

C.   **Nursing Approach**

   1.   Most cross-cultural differences occur because the nurse does not take the time to explore the practice and determine the significance of a practice to the family (Display 12-2).

   2.   A nurse can increase awareness easily if he or she is willing to take the time to become informed and then practice what is learned.

   3.   People want their practices understood and will respect the caregiver who attempts to use their language, inquire with an openness about significant practices, and demonstrates respect for their beliefs.

IV. Major Cultural Groups in the Community

A.   **Hispanic Americans**

   1.   Characteristics

        a.   Half come from Mexico; others come from Puerto Rico, Cuba, Central America

        b.   The fastest growing ethnic group in the United States

DISPLAY 12-2.
Ethnocentric Examples of Community Health Nursing Practice

> ► A new community health nurse, wanting to display friendliness, refers to a group of newly immigrated elderly Southeast Asian refugee women by their first names. This shows disrespect in their culture, and the nurse fails to gain their trust.
> ► A community health nurse visits a family, new to the city, from a rural Appalachian community and instructs them not to give their baby the catnip tea they were using. The nurse was not allowed in the home in the future. This practice was very significant to the family, and they believed without receiving a certain amount of the tea the baby would die. The nurse could have explored the practice with the family, verified its safety with a pharmacist, encouraged formula in an appropriate amount in addition to the tea, and remained a resource to the family.
> ► In a community planning session with a Native-American group, a community health nurse talks during silences and assertively offers solutions. To the group, this is offensive and a sign of immaturity.
> ► When visiting a Mexican-American family, the community health nurse discourages the use of the services offered by an older woman in the community recognized as a local lay healer. He suggests that the family would benefit by visiting the local clinic for health care. The nurse did not recognize the importance of using the "curandero's" suggestions and services. The family followed their familiar ways and would not use the clinic. The nurse could have explored the value of traditional medicine practices and integrated it with the practices he wanted to introduce.

2. Culture
   a. Spanish is a common and primary language with different dialects.
   b. Extended cohesive families are valued.
   c. Families are patriarchal; males are superior (machismo); females (self-sacrificing) bond family life.
   d. Traditional family roles are changing due to urbanization, migration, and women in the work setting.
   e. Religion (Catholicism) plays an important part in the culture.
3. Health beliefs and practices
   a. Cope with illness through prayers and faith that God will heal
   b. Influenced by religious beliefs and some witchcraft
   c. Belief in "hot" and "cold" categories of foods influences diet during illness and after childbirth
4. Health problems
   a. Tuberculosis (especially in those under age 35)
   b. Hypertension
   c. Diabetes
   d. Obesity
   e. Infectious diseases (especially AIDS and pneumonia)
   f. Parasitic infections
   g. Malnutrition
   h. Gastroenteritis
   i. Substance abuse
   j. Accidents and violence

B. Asian Americans
1. Characteristics
    a. Mostly immigrants and refugees from Pacific Rim countries: China, Korea, Japan, Thailand, Laos, the Philippines, Vietnam, Cambodia
    b. Immigrants from China and the Philippines make up the largest Asian groups.
    c. Each group is different and should not be treated or responded to as one group.
2. Culture

    a. **Language, values, and customs are distinctly different.**
    b. Commonalities include patriarchal households with patrilineal lineage; males are valued over females.
    c. Male role—provider; female role—homemaker
    d. Elders are respected.
    e. Saving face or preserving dignity and family pride is very important.
    f. Cooperation is valued over competition.
3. Health beliefs and practices
    a. Vary among cultures
    b. Many Asians believe in the Chinese concepts of Yin and Yang (not referring to temperature but to the opposing forces of the universe regulating normal flow of energy).
    c. Traditional self-care practices include healers such as acupuncturists, herbalists, herb pharmacists, spirit and magic experts, or a shaman; some pray for healing, believing illness is an act of God.
4. Health problems
    a. Tuberculosis
    b. Mental illness (this is considered shameful and may be hidden as long as possible)
    c. Malnutrition
    d. Cancer
    e. Respiratory infections
    f. Chronic diseases associated with aging
    g. Suicide and stress-related illnesses (high among Asian refugee groups)

C. African Americans
1. Characteristics
    a. One third of the population is under 18 years old; over one half of the children live with only their mothers.
    b. The majority of the aged are female.
    c. Social, economic, and educational disparities exist; 50% of prison population is African American; unemployment rates three times higher, lower wages, higher school drop-

out rates, fewer enrolled in or completing college than whites

2. Culture
   a. Because of the diverse countries of origin and size of this group of people, there is no common culture.
   b. The majority of African Americans have absorbed most of the dominant culture in the United States.
   c. Primary language of most African Americans is English.
   d. Many African Americans speak variations of soul talk (black English) or black Creole, which symbolize racial pride and identity.

3. Health beliefs and practices
   a. Many believe health is a sign of harmony with nature and illness is evidence of disharmony.
   b. Disharmony occurs because of evil spirits, God's punishment, or a hex.
   c. Healers treat body, mind, and spirit.
   d. Self-care practices include prayer, laying on of hands, home remedies, magic or other rituals, special diets, wearing preventive charms, using ointments.

4. Health problems
   a. Hypertension
   b. Cardiovascular disease
   c. Cerebral vascular accidents
   d. Cancer
   e. Diabetes mellitus
   f. Cirrhosis
   g. Infant mortality rates twice as high as the white population
   h. Homicide and accidents
   i. Malnutrition
   j. Tuberculosis
   k. AIDS

D. Native Americans

1. Characteristics
   a. A diverse group made up of 270 different tribes
   b. They live in 26 states in the United States with more than half living in Arizona, California, New Mexico, North Carolina, and Oklahoma.
   c. Each tribe (or nation) has its distinct language, beliefs, customs, and rituals.
   d. Native Americans live on reservations (large stretches of land, some as large as small states, federally designated for Indians), rancherias (smaller parcels of land, federally designated for Indians), or among the general population of the United States.

      2. Culture

          a. Value dignity of the individual

          b. Value family and community

          c. Respect for advanced age; elders are the leaders

          d. Respect the environment and live in harmony with nature

          e. Value symbolic arts and crafts

          f. Focus on the present, having little concern for the future

          g. Value generosity and sharing, discourage competition

          h. Integrate religion into everyday life

          i. Value thoughtful speech, practice periods of silence

          j. Value rituals and ceremonies

          k. Value patience

      3. Health beliefs and practices

          a. Treat body and soul as one

          b. Use herbal medicines and traditional healing practices

          c. Health beliefs and practices are influenced by cultural values (present orientation vs future orientation).

          d. The use of the health care delivery system is influenced by a history of government paternalism, feelings of oppression, resentment, and lack of trust toward whites.

      4. Health problems

          a. Tend to be both chronic and socially related

          b. Poor sanitation, crowded housing, and low immunization levels contribute to a variety of communicable diseases

          c. Child health problems include fetal alcohol syndrome (FAS), fetal alcohol effects (FAE), dysentery, impetigo, intestinal infectious diseases, skin diseases, staphylococcal infections, respiratory disease, influenza, and pneumonia.

          d. Adult health problems include tuberculosis, diabetes, obesity, alcoholism, violence, injuries, substance abuse.

V. Transcultural Community Health Nursing

  A. Develop Cultural Self-Awareness

      1. Recognize one's own values, beliefs, and practices that make up one's culture

      2. Complete a cultural self-assessment by analyzing:

          a. Influences from own ethnic/racial background

          b. Own verbal and nonverbal communication patterns

          c. Own cultural values and norms

          d. Own religious beliefs and practices

          e. Own health beliefs and practices

  B. Cultivate Cultural Sensitivity

      1. Recognizes that culturally based values, beliefs, and practices influence people and must be considered

      2. Attempt to understand the clients' points of view

      3. Assess client group's culture (Display 12-3)

DISPLAY 12-3.
A Cultural Assessment

Data are gathered and grouped into six categories:
- Ethnic/racial background
- Language and communication patterns
- Cultural values and norms
- Biocultural factors
- Religious beliefs and practices
- Health beliefs and practices

4. Show respect and patience while learning about other cultures
5. Examine culturally derived health practices

VI. Transcultural Approach to the Nursing Process

A. Assessment
1. People do not have the same health beliefs and values; individualize assessment approach without predetermined expectations
2. Each client requires a careful cultural assessment.
3. Gather assessment data from all people involved: heads of the household, each family member, lay and religious community leaders.
4. Some health beliefs and practices appear to be abusive or to have no effective use; an understanding of the client's belief behind the practice is essential.

B. Planning
1. Each subcultural group has its own set of health beliefs and practices, which must be determined before planning interventions.
2. Effective plans must be made in collaboration with the client, family, or community group.

C. Implementation
1. Implement with the individual's or group's preferences
2. The pace of implementation matches the individual's or group's style of making changes; cultural holidays, beliefs, or events may create a longer implementation phase than expected.

D. Evaluation
1. What is actually implemented may take a different form than the perceived outcome held by the community health nurse; if it works for the client and improves his or her health, it is a positive change.
2. The plan has been implemented; goals have been achieved.
3. The change coexists with cultural practices.

Bibliography

Leininger, M. (1994). *Transcultural nursing: Concepts, theory, research and practice* (2nd ed.). Columbus, OH: McGraw Hill and Greyden Press.

Martin, M. E., & Henry, M. (1989). Cultural relativity and poverty. *Public Health Nursing,* 6(1), 28–34.

Spector, R. E. (1996). *Cultural diversity in health and illness* (4th ed.). Stamford, CT: Appleton & Lange.

Spradley, B. W., & Allender, J. A. (1996). *Community health nursing: Concepts and practice.* (4th ed.). Philadelphia: Lippincott-Raven.

Stanhope, M., & Lancaster, J. (1992). *Community health nursing: Process and practice for promoting health* (3rd ed.). St. Louis: Mosby–Year Book.

West, E. A. (1993). The cultural bridge model. *Nursing Outlook, 41*(5), 229–234.

STUDY QUESTIONS

1. The importance of exploring the diversity among people interacting in the health care arena includes:
   a. A richer understanding of all people delivering and receiving care
   b. A change in the diversity and making it more homogeneous
   c. Improvement in the mix of people to have a balance in the health care system
   d. The alteration of beliefs, opinions, and attitudes that will exist

2. The best definition of *culture* is:
   a. A biologically designated group of people who have distinguishing features
   b. A collection of people with common origins and shared identity
   c. The beliefs, values, and behavior that are shared by members of a society
   d. The variety of patterns that coexist within a geographic area

3. Diversity in the United States includes:
   a. More than ten different ethnic groups living in the country
   b. Immigration patterns that have remained constant over the years
   c. The largest minority group of people being from Cuba
   d. Three minority groups that make up over 45% of the United States

4. Specific gender and age differences that exist in the United States include:
   a. Twice as many male infants than female are born each year
   b. More males than females under age 25 die prematurely
   c. Equal numbers of men and women over age eighty
   d. Cancer affects females over the age of 40 much more than males

5. Ethnocentrism in community health nursing is:
   a. A desired effect to be achieved by the most experienced nurses
   b. An approach to clients that improves their level of wellness
   c. The feeling about one's own culture that inhibits working with diverse groups
   d. An effective way of dealing with people from other cultural groups

6. A community health nurse refers to a group of Southeast Asian elders by their first names, after they have gotten to know the nurse, and the nurse received the permission of the elders. This would be considered:
   a. The right way to approach this group of clients
   b. Ethnocentric and a form of familiarity that should be avoided
   c. Inappropriate to call any elder by a first name
   d. Preferable to remaining formal by using last names

7. Hispanic-American culture and/or characteristics include:
   a. A matriarchal family structure
   b. A common primary language with different dialects
   c. Being independent from extended family members
   d. Fundamentalist Christian beliefs

8. Asian-American culture and/or characteristics include:
   a. Different languages, values, and customs among Asian groups
   b. Competition at school and work being valued over cooperation
   c. English as a primary language, because it is taught in Asian countries
   d. Respecting children and teenagers over elders in various Asian groups

9. African-American culture and/or characteristics include:
   a. A majority of the aged being male
   b. Broad social and economic growth
   c. Low unemployment rates
   d. One third of the population under 18 years old

10. Transcultural nursing and the assessment phase of the nursing process include:

   a. Determining if the goals have been achieved

   b. Pacing the changes to match cultural preferences of the group

   c. Gathering data about cultural beliefs and practices

   d. Collaborating with community members

ANSWER KEY

1. **Correct response: a**
    Answer choices **b, c,** and **d** may or may not be outcome choices. The best choice is a to develop a richer understanding of clients and caregivers. From that understanding, other goals may be desired.
    Comprehension/Psychosocial/Assessment

2. **Correct response: c**
    Answer choice **a** is the definition of *race.*
    Answer choice **b** is the definition of *ethnic group.*
    Answer choice **d** is the definition of *cultural diversity.*
    Knowledge/NA/Assessment

3. **Correct response: d**
    There are more than 100 ethnic groups with immigration patterns that have changed dramatically over the years, and the Cubans are a smaller minority group in the United States.
    Comprehension/NA/Assessment

4. **Correct response: b**
    Answer choices **a, c,** and **d,** are incorrect. A fairly equal number of male and female infants are born each year, there are twice as many women as men over age 80, and cancer affects both sexes in equal numbers but in different sites.
    Comprehension/Health Promotion/Analysis

5. **Correct response: c**
    Answer choices **a, b,** and **d** are incorrect. Being ethnocentric is not a desirable state. Approaching clients with ethnocentric attitudes does not improve their level of wellness and is not an effective way to deal with others.
    Application/Psychosocial/Analysis

6. **Correct response: a**
    Answer choices **b, c,** and **d** are incorrect. Familiarity is not to be avoided; it depends on the individual. It is only inappropriate to call someone by a first name if they prefer not to be addressed that way. Using last names is appropriate initially and preferable if it is the client choice.
    Application/Safe Care/Implementation

7. **Correct response: b**
    Hispanic family structure is patriarchal. Hispanics have cohesive extended families and are predominantly Catholic.
    Comprehension/Safe Care/Analysis

8. **Correct response: a**
    Asian Americans value cooperation over competition, have many native languages that remain primary in immigrant groups, and respect elders.
    Comprehension/Safe Care/Analysis

9. **Correct response: d**
    The majority of the aged are female, social and economic problems exist without significant growth, and unemployment rates are high.
    Comprehension/Safe Care/Analysis

10. **Correct response: c**
    Answer choice **a** is from the evaluation phase, **b** is the implementation phase, and **d** is from the planning phase.
    Application/Safe Care/Evaluation

Community Health Nurses: Assessing Healthy Families

I. Characteristics of Families

A. Definitions

1. A family is who the members say it is.
2. One or more individuals who share a residence, or live near one another, possess some common emotional bond, and engage in interrelated social positions, roles, and tasks (Spradley & Allender, 1996).
3. Two or more individuals coming from the same or different kinship groups who are involved in a continuous living arrangement, usually residing in the same household, experi-

encing common emotional bonds, and sharing certain obliga-
tions toward each other and toward others (Stanhope &
Lancaster, 1992).

B.   Structures

    1.   Traditional

        a.   Nuclear family: father, mother, and children living in the
same household

        b.   Single-adult family: single adult living alone either by
choice or because of separation, divorce, or death

        c.   Multigenerational family: several generations or age
groups living together in the same household

        d.   Kin-network family: several nuclear families living in the
same household, or near one another, and sharing goods
and services (frequently seen in close-knit ethnic communities)

        e.   Blended family: divorced or widowed parents marrying
and raising the children from each of their previous mar-
riages

        f.   Single-parent family: one adult caring for a child or chil-
dren as a result of separation, divorce, death, or by choice

        g.   Commuter family: both parents working, but their jobs
are in different cities, with a "home" city, where one parent works and the family lives, and the other parent com-
mutes and is home on weekends

    2.   Nontraditional

        a.   Cohabitating couple: adults of all ages sharing their lives
outside of the bonds of marriage for a variety of reasons

        b.   Commune family: a group of unrelated, monogamous
couples living together and collectively rearing their children

        c.   Group-marriage family: several adults sharing a common
household who consider that all are married to each
other, sharing everything including sex and child rearing

        d.   Group-network family: nuclear families bound by a com-
mon set of values living close to each other and sharing
goods, services, and child-rearing responsibilities

        e.   Foster family: family accepting unrelated children into the
home on a temporary basis while the parent(s) receive the
necessary help to reunite the original family

        f.   Homeless family: families finding themselves without per-
manent shelter due to personal crises often related to
negative economic changes and/or chronic mental health
problems

        g.   Gang: a destructive family form made up of young people
searching for the emotional ties of a close and caring family, but engaging in violence and crime as a way of life

    C.   Functions
- 1. Affection
  - a. Establish a climate of affection
  - b. Promote sexuality and sexual fulfillment
  - c. Add new members
- 2. Security and acceptance
  - a. Maintain physical requirements
  - b. Accept individual members
- 3. Identity and satisfaction
  - a. Maintain motivation
  - b. Develop self-image and role
  - c. Identify social placement and satisfying activities
- 4. Affiliation and companionship
  - a. Develop communication patterns
  - b. Establish durable bonds
- 5. Socialization
  - a. Internalize culture (values and behavior)
  - b. Guide internal and external relationships
  - c. Release members
- 6. Controls
  - a. Maintain social control
  - b. Divide labor
  - c. Allocate and use resources

II. **Duvall's Eight Stages of the Family Life Cycle (Fig. 13-1)**

III. **Emerging Family Patterns**

    A.   Divorce (Table 13-1)

    B.   Remarriage and Blending Families (Table 13-2)
- 1. Many people do not remarry after divorce and choose to remain single, regardless of age or circumstance at the time of divorce.
- 2. Some people postpone blending families through remarriage until children are grown. The new union, however, affects all concerned in different ways, no matter what age.

IV. **Family Health Assessment**

    A.   Guidelines
- 1. Focus on the family as a total unit.
- 2. Ask goal-directed questions.
- 3. Collect data over time.
- 4. Combine quantitative and qualitative data.
- 5. Exercise professional judgment.

    B.   **Data Collection: gather data on family structure, functions and development; format varies to meet organizational needs (Display 13-1)**
- 1. Questionnaires
  - a. Detailed questions placed on a form and completed by the nurse with checks, words, or short phrases

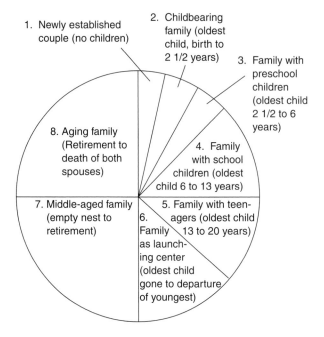

FIGURE 13–1.
Duvall's eight stages of the nuclear family life cycle. Size of wedge reflects relative percent of total life cycle spent in each stage.

      b.   Ideally, the information is gathered in a casual, conversational manner.

      c.   Can be lengthy and time consuming to complete

    d.   **The nurse may focus on the form and not the family.**

   2.   Open-ended family assessments

      a.   The nurse asks open-ended questions aimed at determining family health.

TABLE 13-1.
Phases of a Family Divorce

PHASE	TIME FRAME
Stressors leading to marital difference	May have existed since before the marriage
Decision to divorce	Years to weeks
Planning dissolution of the family system	Months to weeks
Separation	Years or not at all
Divorce	Day(s) in court—hours to minutes
Post-divorce	Persons recover in their own timeframe (most likely 1 year to several years)

TABLE 13-2.
Phases of Remarriage and Blending Families

PHASE	TIMEFRAME
Meeting new people	Begins in the postdivorce phase and continues indefinitely
Entering a new relationship	To have an effective relationship, need to have completed an "emotional recovery" from past divorce—1 year to years
Planning a new marriage	Months to years—depends on new roles, responsibilities, finances, children
Remarriage and blending of families	It takes work to blend two families. Success may only be achieved after years

   b.   Questions need to be phrased in lay terms in order for families to understand the meaning (when asking about internal resources or strengths, the question may be "What keeps you going or motivates you?" or "What are some of your best features?").
3.   Videotaping family interactions
   a.   Suggested by a community health nurse with the technical skills to use the needed equipment and the counseling skills necessary to effectively analyze the findings with the family
   b.   With family permission and an explanation of the purpose
   c.   View the tape with the family and pause at times to discuss your observations and the family members' observations and reactions.
   d.   Use the reactions and responses to develop a plan for change.

DISPLAY 13-1.
Data Collection Categories

Family demographics
Physical environment
Psychological and spiritual environment
Family structure/roles
Family values and beliefs
Family communication patterns
Family decision-making patterns
Family problem-solving patterns
Family coping patterns
Family health behavior
Family social and cultural patterns

    e. A follow-up video demonstrating the change can be compared with the original as part of the evaluation phase of the nursing process.

    f. An especially good tool to monitor changes in parenting skills, family communication patterns

4. Structured observations

    a. The nurse observes family interactions using a tool that consists of a ranking of observed behaviors.

    b. This information gives the nurse quantitative data of the quality of family interaction.

    c. With this information, the nurse collaborates with the family on recommendations.

5. Analysis of life-changing events

    a. Uses scales depicting stressors in families and the potential effects

    b. Used to help families identify sources of stress in their lives

    c. This information assists with life planning.

    d. A classic tool—Holmes and Rahe Social Readjustment Rating Scale, 1967

C. Methods

1. Eco-map

    a. Diagrams the connections between a family and the other systems in its ecologic environment

    b. Involves family members in the map's development

    c. Depicts the family by a large circle in the center with smaller circles on the periphery to represent significant people and systems

    d. Connects the circles with different style lines depicting the quality of the relationship

    e. Stimulates discussion and analysis of relationships

2. Genogram

    a. Displays complex family patterns

    b. Becomes a rich source of family information over generations

    c. Diagrams family relationships by listing the family genealogy accompanied by significant life events

    d. Serves as a tool used jointly with the family; encourages family expression

    e. Sheds light on family behavior and problems

3. Social network support map

    a. Gives detail regarding the quality and quantity of social connections in a map or grid

    b. Elaborates the strengths within the system through words, checks, and/or numbers

      c.   Serves as a tool to help the family understand its sources of support and relationships

      d.   Forms a basis for nursing care planning and intervention

V.   Individual Health Assessments:

m **Developmental—used to collect standard data on clients as a baseline; promotes continuity of care and quality assurance**

  A.   Child

      1.   Newborn Checklist

         a.   Developed by agencies to document home or clinic visits

         b.   Initiated on a first visit after birth

         c.   Provides baseline and continuing visit information

         d.   Includes appropriate infant parameters needing assessment during the first year of life

      2.   Denver II—DDST—The Denver Developmental Screening Test (2nd ed., 1992)

         a.   Considered a classic tool with demonstrated reliability and validity for community health nurses since 1967

         b.   Used to assess developmental task accomplishment in children from birth to age 6

         c.   Used by the nurse to teach the family activities that will promote age-appropriate development or to make referrals as necessary

         d.   Conducted with the assistance of the child's caregiver (15- to 20-minute test)

         e.   Must be administered exactly as instructed by the manual or can skew results

      3.   PDQ—The Pre-Denver Questionnaire

         a.   A ten-item questionnaire asked of the child's caregiver

         b.   If there are two or more "no" responses, a DDST test is performed on the child.

         c.   Considered a good screening device that takes 1 to 2 minutes and does not need the child's participation; can be administered by paraprofessionals

      4.   Healthy Child Scale

         a.   Developed by the agency as a visit documentation tool for gathering baseline and continued visit information

         b.   Initiated when a family case is opened

         c.   Documents age-appropriate major growth and developmental tasks, height, weight, immunizations, history of illnesses and accidents, names of health care professionals

  B.   Adult

      1.   Well Adult Scale

         a.   Developed by agencies as a visit documentation tool for gathering baseline and continued visit information

         b.   Initiated when a family case is opened

        c.   Documents age-appropriate major growth and developmental tasks, height, weight, immunizations, history of illnesses and accidents, names of health care professionals

2. Prenatal Checklist
- a. Developed by agencies to document home or clinic visits
- b. Initiated on a first visit
- c. Provides baseline and continued visit information
- d. Includes prenatal information needing assessment at different trimesters throughout pregnancy

3. Postpartum Checklist
- a. Developed by agencies to document home or clinic visits
- b. Initiated on a first visit after delivery
- c. Provides a form with baseline and continued visit information
- d. Includes postpartum information needing assessment for 6 weeks after delivery

C. Disease

    1. Chronic Checklist
- a. Developed by agencies to document visits to individuals with chronic illnesses
- b. Initiated on a first visit by the community health nurse
- c. Provides baseline and continued visit information
- d. Includes disease entity information needing assessment during the caregiving; includes signs, symptoms, appropriate teaching, referrals, other pertinent information to enhance continuity of care
- e. Examples include diabetes, congestive heart failure (CHF), chronic obstructive pulmonary disease (COPD), arterial sclerotic heart disease (ASHD), renal failure, hypertension

    2. Acute Checklist
- a. Developed by agencies to document visits to individuals with acute illnesses
- b. Initiated on the first visit by the community health nurse
- c. Provides baseline and continued visit documentation
- d. Includes disease entity information needing assessment during caregiving; includes signs, symptoms, appropriate teaching, referrals, other pertinent information to enhance continuity of care
- e. Examples include surgeries, injuries, infections, communicable diseases

D. Nutrition: The Food Pyramid Guide (Fig. 13-2)

    1. Used as a basic standard with which to conduct nutritional assessments

    2. Modified based on culture, age, weight, pregnancy, specific diseases

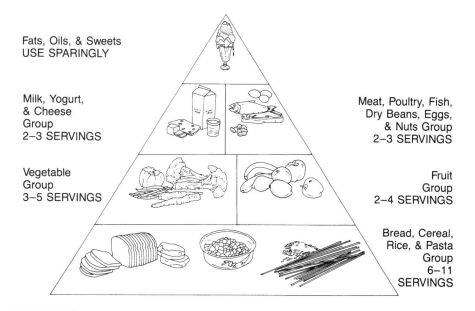

Fats, Oils, & Sweets
USE SPARINGLY

Milk, Yogurt,
& Cheese
Group
2–3 SERVINGS

Meat, Poultry, Fish,
Dry Beans, Eggs,
& Nuts Group
2–3 SERVINGS

Vegetable
Group
3–5 SERVINGS

Fruit
Group
2–4 SERVINGS

Bread, Cereal,
Rice, & Pasta
Group
6–11
SERVINGS

FIGURE 13-2.
The Food Guide Pyramid. In April of 1992, the U.S. Department of Agriculture replaced the old four food groups, in use since 1946, with the Food Pyramid. It emphasizes grains, fruits, and vegetables as the basis of a healthy diet. Recommended daily servings in each group are noted.

VI. Family Health
A. Characteristics
1. There is healthy interaction among family members.
2. The family enhances individual development.
3. Their role relationships are structured effectively.
4. The family actively attempts to cope with problems.
5. They have a healthy home environment and lifestyle.
6. They establish regular links with the broader community.

B. Levels of Prevention
1. Primary
   a. Adults are well prepared for the responsibilities of marriage and parenthood.
   b. Adults enter parenthood with the personal resource necessary to promote the growth and development of the family unit.
2. Secondary
   a. Early recognition of problems in the relationships among or between family members, the family seeks out appropriate resources
   b. If one family member has personal problems (which can affect the family as a whole), appropriate resources are sought out.

        c.   Activities at this level bring the family to the highest level of wellness possible.

    3.   Tertiary

        a.   After the family suffers a crisis, the members recognize the need for help, seek it out, and accept that help.

        b.   Families draw on personal resources to rebuild relationships and heal the family unit.

        c.   Activities at this level bring the family to the highest level of wellness possible.

C.   **Effects of Unhealthy Families on the Community**

    1.   Unhealthy family structures have members who have learning and behavior difficulties, mental health problems, chemical dependency, family violence.

    2.   Poorly functioning families drain community resources; the police system, child welfare services, educational systems.

    3.   Violence spills out of the family and into the community: crimes against persons, property, or possessions escalate; communities suffer; the nation suffers.

VII.   **The Nursing Process in Family Assessment**

   A.   **Assessment**

    1.   Know who makes up the family; each person's role; authority patterns

    2.   Base plans on an analysis of family strengths

   B.   **Planning**

    1.   Start where the family is

    2.   Work with the family collectively

   C.   **Implementation**

    1.   Adapt nursing intervention to the family's stage of development

    2.   Recognize the validity of family structural variations

    3.   Emphasize family strengths

   D.   **Evaluation**

    1.   Summarize family strengths, resources, areas needing intervention

    2.   Assess the extent that the expected outcomes were met based on knowledge about the family

    3.   Reassess family if goals are not met

Bibliography

Duvall, E. M., & Miller, B. (1985). *Marriage and family development* (6th ed.). New York: Harper & Row.

Frankenburg, W. K., & Dodds, J. B. (1992) *Denver II.* Denver, CO: Denver Developmental Materials.

Holmes, T., & Rahe, T. (1967). The social readjustment rating scale. *Journal of Psychosomatic Research, 11,* 213–217.

Spradley, B. W., & Allender, J. A. (1996). *Community health nursing: Concepts and practice.* (4th ed.). Philadelphia: Lippincott-Raven.

Stanhope, M., & Lancaster, J. (1992). *Community health nursing: Process and practice for promoting health.* (3rd ed.). St. Louis: Mosby–Year Book.

STUDY QUESTIONS

1. All definitions of a family include the following thoughts and expectations:
   a. A married couple with or without children
   b. Individuals who share a residence and have common emotional bonds .
   c. People related by bloodlines, no matter where they live
   d. A single person living alone with no significant others in their life

2. Identify which of the following family structures represent a nontraditional family.
   a. Nuclear family
   b. Multigenerational family
   c. Cohabitating couple
   d. Single-parent families

3. This is a destructive family form made up of young people searching for a close and caring family, but who engage in violence and crime as a way of life.
   a. Commune families
   b. Foster families
   c. Homeless families
   d. Gang families

4. Emerging family patterns include:
   a. Divorced and blended families
   b. Group-network families
   c. Group-marriage families
   d. Commuter families

5. When conducting a family assessment, the community health nurse:
   a. Focuses on the most ill family member
   b. Asks questions that are closed, to get precise information
   c. Focuses on data that can be quantified
   d. Collects data over time from all family members

6. A variety of assessment methods are used to collect family data. When the nurse develops a display of complex family patterns, which diagrams family relationships through generations, the nurse has developed a(n):
   a. Eco-map
   b. Genogram
   c. Social network support map
   d. Gantt chart

7. The purpose of completing a family assessment is to:
   a. Help the family understand its sources of support
   b. Gather data on family structure, function, and development
   c. Encourage family expression on family behavior and problems
   d. Discuss and analyze relationships

8. An individual assessment tool that involves the assessment of the growth and developmental tasks of children from birth through age 6 is:
   a. The Holmes and Rahe Scale
   b. Videotaping family interaction
   c. The Denver Developmental Screening Test
   d. The Food Pyramid Guide

9. Characteristics of a healthy family include:
   a. Role relationships that are unstructured
   b. Remaining separate from the broader community
   c. Coping with problems through avoidance
   d. Enhancing individual development

10. In a healthy family, adults are well prepared for the responsibilities of marriage and parenthood. This is an example of:
    a. Primary prevention
    b. Secondary prevention
    c. Tertiary prevention
    d. Blended family

ANSWER KEY

1. *Correct response: b*
   Answer choice **a** assumes one must be married to be considered a family, choice **c** implies a family needs to be related by bloodlines, and in choice **d** the person meets none of the characteristics of a family, as included in answer choice **b.**
   Comprehension/Psychosocial/Analysis

2. *Correct response: c*
   Answer choices **a, b,** and **d** represent family structure types that have been traditional in the United States. It is more recently that cohabitating people have been considered an example of a nontraditional family.
   Knowledge/NA/Assessment

3. *Correct response: d*
   Answer choices **a, b,** and **c** depict examples of nontraditional families. The gang family is also nontraditional.
   Knowledge/NA/Assessment

4. *Correct response: a*
   Answer choices **b** and **c** are examples of nontraditional families. Choice **d** is an example of a traditional family. Emerging are large numbers of divorced families, remarriages, and a blending of families.
   Comprehension/Psychosocial/Analysis

5. *Correct response: d*
   Answer choice **a** indicates there is an ill family member in the household; visits may be to healthy families.
   Choice **b**—ask questions that are open-ended and goal directed.
   Choice **c**—data need to be quantitative and qualitative.
   Application/Safe Care/Implementation

6. *Correct response: b*
   Answer choices **a** and **c** are other assessment methods.

   Choice **d** is a time-line chart used in planning within agencies (see Chap. 6).
   Comprehension/Safe Care/Analysis

7. *Correct response: b*
   Answer choice **a** describes the specific function of the social network support map.
   Answer choice **c** describes the specific function of the genogram.
   Choice **d** describes the function of the eco-map.
   Application/Safe Care/Implementation

8. *Correct response: c*
   Answer choice **a** is a social readjustment rating scale.
   Choice **b** is another form of gathering family assessment data.
   Choice **d** is a model for food intake (quantity and type of food).
   Comprehension/Safe Care/Analysis

9. *Correct response: d*
   Answer choice **a**—in healthy families, role relationships are structured effectively.
   Choice **b**—the healthy family establishes regular links with the broader community.
   Choice **c**—the healthy family actively attempts to cope with problems.
   Comprehension/Safe Care/Assessment

10. *Correct response: a*
    Being well prepared for marriage and parenthood establishes a healthy family at a level of prevention that is the most beneficial and least costly in terms of stress and use of resources. A blended family may or may not be healthy.
    Analysis/Safe Care/Evaluation

Improving the Health of Aggregates in the Community

I. Healthy People 2000

    A. Broad Goals

        1. Increase the span of healthy life for Americans
        2. Reduce health disparities among Americans
        3. Achieve access to preventive services for all Americans

    B. Objectives: This government document contains a national prevention strategy for improving the health of the citizens of the United States during the 1990 to 2000 decade.

        1. Health professionals from numerous disciplines, health advocates, and consumers contributed to formulating objectives for the document.

2. The document contains norms for health conditions and identifies major health topics and areas for the year 2000.

3. The document organizes 300 specific objectives into 22 priority areas under the broad categories of health promotion, health protection, and preventive services.

II. Maternal and Infant Health

A. Specific Needs

1. (Potential) maternal population

   a. Females need to be able to decide when pregnancy will occur, if they are sexually active.

   b. Females need to have family planning methods that are affordable and accessible.

   c. Pregnancy should be postponed until the parent(s) can provide for the infant emotionally, physically, and financially.

   d. Accessible and adequate prenatal care should include education that encourages abstinence from drugs and alcohol during pregnancy and other behaviors that ensure a full-term delivery.

   e. An informed delivery and adequate hospital stay may promote entrance into an uneventful postpartum period.

   f. Postpartal care should include an effective family planning method of choice.

   g. The employer should consider the needs of the woman, by providing adequate maternity leave and infant care services when she returns to work.

2. Infants in the first year of life

   a. A safe birthing process promotes a healthy start in life.

   b. Breastfeeding is recommended for nutrition and bonding.

   c. An infant needs adequate love, nutrition, stimulation, sleep, health care, and immunizations, in a safe living environment (Display 14-1)

B. Goals of Healthy People 2000: Selected Objectives for Maternal and Infant Population (Display 14-2)

C. Levels of Prevention

1. Primary

   a. Teach measures (healthy living habits, immunizations, and safety practices) to keep illness or injury from ever occurring in maternal–infant population

   b. Pregnancy: proper diet, rest, and exercise; prenatal care; avoiding infectious diseases, drugs, and alcohol

   c. Postpartum: proper diet, rest, and exercise; postpartum visits; select a family planning method; prepare for a possible "let down" emotionally; plan to return to normal activities including work and recreation

    d.   Infant: proper care, which includes nutrition (how to breastfeed successfully), sleep, cleanliness, safety, stimulation, immunizations and well baby health care practitioner visits, safe living environment, knowledgeable caregivers (especially if mother is returning to work), love

  2. Secondary

    a.   Screening procedures; early diagnosis to detect, diagnose, and treat abnormalities (hemoglobin, red blood count, sexually transmitted diseases [STDs]) at the earliest possible stage to encourage a return to wellness

    b.   Pregnancy and postpartum: early detection of signs and symptoms of infection, premature labor, depression; immediate and proper care when variations from normal are first detected

    c.   Infant: early detection of signs and symptoms of illness or injury; receive immediate and proper health care when variations from normal growth and development or wellness state are first detected; problem solve difficult breastfeeding patterns

  3. Tertiary

    a.   Attempt to reduce the extent and severity of conditions related to pregnancy (pregnancy-induced hypertension [PIH], diabetes, injury) by initiating rehabilitation to minimize effects on the fetus and preserve the pregnancy

    b.   Pregnancy: treat the condition to preserve the pregnancy, induce labor, terminate the pregnancy if the mother's life is threatened; if viable—cesarean delivery

    c.   Postpartum: treat irregular lochia patterns, depression, infections; cesarean incision healing; returning to normal activities

    d.   Infant: follow health care practitioner recommendations for care, seek help from others (family and friends) as needed, prevent further complications

D. **Selected Skills of the Community Health Nurse (see Chap. 5)**

  1. Advocate

    a.   Speak out for the clients; cut "red-tape" to assist in receiving appropriate maternal–infant services

    b.   Take broad concerns to the appropriate problem solver; local, state, or federal level; speak professionally on behalf of needed changes

  2. Case manager

    a.   Assess, plan, and coordinate maternal–infant services; refer to appropriate providers

    b.   Monitor and evaluate response to services to ensure that needs are met emotionally, physically, and financially

text continued on page 180

DISPLAY 14-1.
American Academy of Pediatrics Committee on Infectious Diseases

Recommended Childhood Immunization Schedule—United States, January–December 1997

The American Academy of Pediatrics (AAP) has harmonized the Recommended Childhood Immunization Schedule with the Advisory Committee on Immunization Practices (ACIP) of the Centers for Disease Control and Prevention (CDC) and the American Academy of Family Physicians (AAFP) since January 1995. Since the last schedule was issued in July 1996,[1] the following developments with resulting changes in immunization recommendations have occurred:

1. As of early 1997, the recommendations for polio immunization in the United States have been revised. The complete AAP policy statement for the use of inactivated poliovirus vaccine (IPV) and oral poliovirus vaccine (OPV) will be published concurrently or in an upcoming issue of *Pediatrics*. Each of the following schedules is acceptable by the AAP, the ACIP, and the AAFP: (1) *sequential:* IPV at 2 and 4 months, OPV at 12 to 18 months, and 4 to 6 years, (2) *IPV only:* IPV at 2, 4, 12 to 18 months, and 4 to 6 years, (3) *OPV only:* OPV at 2, 4, 6 to 18 months, and 4 to 6 years. Parents and providers may choose among these schedules. The ACIP recommends the sequential schedule for most children. IPV is the only poliovirus vaccine recommended for immunocompromised persons and their household contacts.

2. As of December 5, 1996, one acellular pertussis vaccine combined with diphtheria and tetanus toxiods (DTaP) (Tripedia, Connaught Laboratories, Swiftwater, PA) was ap-

5. Other new combination products that are licensed by the FDA may be used whenever administration of components of the vaccine are indicated. The package inserts should be consulted for details.

6. The footnotes for DTaP/DTP, poliovirus, and Hib vaccines have been modified to take into account these recent developments. Other changes have been made in the hepatitis B, measles, and varicella footnotes to clarify recommendations. Of particular note, hepatitis B immunization can begin at any age for children who were not immunized in infancy.

COMMITTEE ON INFECTIOUS DISEASES, 1996 to 1997
Neal A. Halsey, MD, Chairperson
Jon S. Abramson, MD
P. Joan Chesney, MD
Margaret C. Fisher, MD
Michael A. Gerber, MD
Donald S. Gromisch, MD
Steve Kohl, MD
S. Michael Marcy, MD
Dennis L. Murray, MD
Gary D. Overturf, MD
Richard J. Whitley, MD
Ram Yogev, MD

proved by the Food and Drug Administration (FDA) for use in infants. DTaP is preferred for use at all ages, but whole-cell pertussis vaccines (DTP) are acceptable alternatives. FDA approval of additional DTaP products for use in infants is anticipated before the 1998 schedule is issued next January.

3. A new combination of DTaP with a conjugate *Haemophilus influenzae* type b (Hib) vaccine (Tripedia-ActHIB) has been approved only for administration as the fourth dose in the DTaP/DTP series for children 15 months of age and older. As of November 15, 1996, this combination was not approved for use in the primary series in infants.

4. A new combination product (COMVAX, Merck, West Point, PA) of hepatitis B and *Haemophilus influenzae* type b (Hib) vaccines has been approved for immunization at 2, 4, and 12 to 15 months of age. This and other Hib-containing vaccines should not be administered to infants younger than 6 weeks. The Hib component administered at earlier ages is not adequately immunogenic and could have an adverse effect on the immune response to subsequent doses of Hib vaccines administered at older ages.

The recomendations in this statement do not indicate an exclusive course of treatment or serve as a standard of medical care. Variations, taking into account individual circumstances, may be appropriate. PEDIATRICS (ISSN 0031 4005). Copyright © 1997 by the American Academy of Pediatrics.

EX-OFFICIO
Georges Peter, MD

LIAISON REPRESENTATIVES
Robert Breiman, MD
  National Vaccine Program Office
M. Carolyn Hardegree, MD
  Food and Drug Administration
Stephen Hadler, MD
  National Immunization Program
Richard F. Jacobs, MD
  American Thoracic Society
Noni E. MacDonald, MD
  Canadian Paediatric Society
Walter A. Orenstein, MD
  National Immunization Program
N. Regina Rabinovich, MD
  National Institutes of Allergy and Infectious Diseases
Ben Schwartz, MD
  Centers for Disease Control and Prevention

REFERENCE

1. American Academy of pediatrics, Committee on Infectious Diseases, Recommended childhood immunization schedule. *Pediatrics* 1996;98:158-160.

DISPLAY 14-1. (continued)

Recommended Childhood Immunization Schedule United States, January–December 1997

Vaccines[1] are listed under the routinely recommended ages. Bars indicate range of acceptable ages for vaccination. Shaded bars indicate catch-up vaccination: at 11–12 years of age, hepatitis B vaccine should be administered to children not previously vaccinated, and Varicella vaccine should be administered to children not previously vaccinated who lack a reliable history of chickenpox.

Age ▶ / Vaccine ▼	Birth	1 mo	2 mos	4 mos	6 mos	12 mos	15 mos	18 mos	4-6 yrs	11-12 yrs	14-16 yrs
Hepatitis B[2,3]	Hep B-1	Hep B-2			Hep B-3					Hep B[3]	
Diphtheria, Tetanus, Pertussis[4]			DTaP or DTP	DTaP or DTP	DTaP or DTP		DTaP or DTP[4]		DTaP or DTP	Td	
H. influenzae type b[5]			Hib	Hib	Hib[5]	Hib[5]					
Polio[6]			Polio[6]	Polio		Polio[6]			Polio		
Measles, Mumps, Rubella[7]						MMR			MMR[7]	or MMR[7]	
Varicella[8]						Var				Var[6]	

Approved by the Advisory Committee on Immunization Practices (ACIP), the American Academy of Pediatrics (AAP), and the American Academy of Family Physicians (AAFP).

[1]This schedule indicates the recommended age for routine administration of currently licensed childhood vaccines. Some combination vaccines are available and may be used whenever administration of all components of the vaccine is indicated. Providers should consult the manufacturers' package inserts for detailed recommendations.

[2]*Infants born to HBsAg-negative mothers* should receive 2.5 μg of Merck vaccine (Recombivax HB) or 10 μg of SmithKline Buecham (SB) vaccine (Engerix-B). The 2nd dose should be administered ≥ 1 mo after the 1st dose.

Infants born to HBsAG-positive mothers should receive 0.5 mL hepatitis B immune globulin (HBIG) within 12 hrs of birth, and either 5 μg of Merck vaccine (Recombivax HB) or 10 μg of SB vaccine (Engerix-B) at a separate site. The 2nd dose is recommended at 1-2 mos of age and the 3rd dose at 6 mos of age.

Infants born to mothers whose HBsAG status is unknown should receive either 5 μg of Merck vaccine (Flecombivax HB) or 10 μg of SB vaccine (Engerix-B) within 12 hrs of birth. The 2nd dose of vaccine is recommended at 1 mo of age and the 3rd dose at 6 mos of age. Blood should be drawn at the time of delivery to determine the mother's HBsAG status; if it is positive, the infant should receive HBIG as soon as possible (no later than 1 wk of age). The dosage and timing of subsequent vaccine doses should be based upon the mother's HBsAG status.

[3]Children and adolescents who have not been vaccinated against hepatitis B in infancy may begin the series during any childhood visit. Those who have not previously received 3 doses of hepatitis B vaccine should initiate or complete the series during the 11–12 year-old visit. The 2nd dose should be administered at least 1 mo after the 1st dose, and the 3rd dose should be administered at least 4 mos after the 1st dose and at least 2 mos after the 2nd dose.

[4]DTaP (diphtheria and tetanus toxoids and acellular pertussis vaccine) is the preferred vaccine for all doses in the vaccination series, including comple-

tion of the series in children who have received ≥1 dose of whole-cell DTP vaccine. Whole-cell DTP is an acceptable alternative to DTaP. The 4th dose of DTaP may be administered as early as 12 months of age, provided 6 months have elapsed since the 3rd dose, and if the child is considered unlikely to return at 15–18 mos of age. Td (tetanus and diphtheria toxoids, absorbed, for adult use) is recommended at 11–12 years of age if at least 5 years have elapsed since the last dose of DTP, DTaP, or DT. Subsequent routine Td boosters are recommended every 10 years.

[5]Three *H. influenzae* type b (Hib) conjugate vaccines are licensed for infant use. If PAP-OMP (PadvaxHIB [Merck]) is administered at 2 and 4 mos of age, a dose at 6 mos is not required. After completing the primary series, any Hib conjugate vaccine may be used as a booster.

[6]Two poliovirus vaccines are currently licensed in the US: inactivated poliovirus vaccine (IPV) and oral poliovirus vaccine (OPV). The following schedules are all acceptable by the ACIP, the AAP, and the AAFP, and parents and providers may choose among them:

   1. IPV at 2 and 4 mos; OPV at 12–18 mos and 4–6 yr
   2. IPV AT 2, 4, 12–18 Mos, and 4–6 yr
   3. OPV at 2, 4, 6–18 mos, and 4–6 yr

The ACIP routinely recommends schedule 1. IPV is the only poliovirus vaccine recommended for immunocompromised persons and their household contacts.

[7]The 2nd dose of MMR is routinely recommended at 4–6 yrs of age or at 11–12 yrs of age, but may be administered during any visit, provided at least 1 month has elapsed since receipt of the 1st dose and that both doses are administered at or after 12 months of age.

[8]Susceptible children may receive Varicella vaccine (Var) at any visit after the first birthday, and those who lack a reliable history of chickenpox should be immunized during the 11–12 year-old visit. Children ≥ 13 years of age should receive 2 doses, at least 1 mos apart.

DISPLAY 14-2.
Selected Maternal and Infant Population Objectives

OBJECTIVE	1987	1990	2000 TARGET
Reduce maternal mortality rate to no more than 3.3 per 100,000 live births	6.6	8.2	3.3
Reduce the cesarean delivery rate to no more than 15 per 100 deliveries	24.4	23.5	15.0
Reduce the infant mortality rate to no more than 7 deaths per 1,000 live births	10.1	9.2	7.0
Reduce the black infant mortality rate to no more than 11 deaths per 1,000 live births	17.9	17.0	11.0
Reduce low birth weight to an incidence of no more than 5% of all live births	6.9	7.0	5.0
Reduce low birth weight to an incidence of no more than 9% of black live births	12.7	13.3	9.0

3. Clinician
   a. Holistic practice: the expanding family has a broad range of interacting needs that affect the collective health of the "client" as a larger system
   b. Focus on wellness: promote health and prevention of illness in maternal–infant population
   c. Expanded skills: with this population, skills are broad; environmental concerns, substance abuse and mental health counseling, anticipatory guidance, social needs, limited funding for maternal–infant programs, collaboration with consumers, professionals, community organizations
4. Collaborator: work with consumers of health care, community members, professionals
5. Counselor: listen to clients and assist them in identifying internal resources; work with community members to identify and meet needs
6. Educator

   a. **Greatest role (in time and talent) with the maternal–infant population**
   b. Teach clients how to promote a healthy pregnancy
7. Researcher
   a. Consumer: remain up-to-date on changes in maternal–infant care practice; use this information to change practice and promote quality and effectiveness
   b. Producer: seeks opportunities to conduct research alone or in collaboration with others to enhance the knowledge base in the field of maternal–infant health

III. Toddler, Preschool, School Age, and Adolescent Health

A. Specific Needs

1. Growth and development will proceed successfully uninterrupted by delays enhanced by parents who provide a safe and stimulating environment.
2. The child should be nurtured in a safe environment and will grow and develop the skills to make informed decisions and healthy relationships that will prepare for adulthood.
3. The child will receive appropriate immunizations, screening, and health education to promote a high level of wellness.
4. Formal and informal educational processes are supported by the community and family to prepare the child for a productive and satisfying adulthood.

B. Goals of Healthy People 2000: Selected Objectives for the Toddler, Preschool, School Age, and Adolescent Population (Display 14-3)

C. Levels of Prevention

1. Primary

 a. **Teach healthy living habits to keep illness or injury from ever occurring in the child and youth population, especially accident prevention, the leading cause of death in children**

   b. Make immunizations accessible (physically and financially) to all children and youth (see Display 14-1)

   c. Provide parents with anticipatory guidance to prepare child adequately for increasing independence

DISPLAY 14-3.
Selected Objectives—Toddler, Preschool, School Age, and Adolescent Population

OBJECTIVE	1987 BASELINE	2000 TARGET
Reduce the death rate for children to no more than 28 per 100,000 children aged 1 through 14	33	28
Reduce deaths among children age 14 and younger caused by motor vehicle crashes to no more than 5.5 per 100,000	6.2	5.5
Reduce the initiation of cigarette smoking by children and youth so no more than 15% have become a cigarette smoker by age 20	30	20
Enact in 50 states laws requiring that new handguns be designed to minimize the likelihood of discharge by children	0	50
Reduce the death rate for adolescents and young adults to no more than 85 per 100,000	99.4	85

       d.   Instruct parents to keep channels of communication open with the child and the systems in which the child interacts

  2. Secondary

       a.   Early diagnosis and treatment: identified through screening procedures to detect, diagnose, and treat age-related health concerns (lead levels, vision and hearing, scoliosis, STDs, abuse, violence) at the earliest possible stage to encourage a return to wellness

       b.   Prompt treatment of injuries related to falls, crashes, or violence that occurs at play, on bicycles, motor vehicles, or from violence at home or in the community

  3. Tertiary

       a.   Initiate rehabilitation to minimize effects on the child; return to the highest level of wellness; in some cases to extend and save a child's life

       b.   Attempt to reduce the extent and severity of an illness; ear infections, tonsillitis, asthma, substance use, depression, cancers

       c.   Attempt to reduce the extent and severity of injuries; wounds, broken bones, internal injuries

D. **Selected Skills of the Community Health Nurse**

  1. Advocate

       a.   Speak out for the clients; cut "red-tape" to receive appropriate child health services

       b.   Take broad child health concerns to the appropriate problem solver; local, state, or federal level; speak professionally on behalf of needed changes

  2. Case manager

       a.   Assess, plan, and coordinate child health services; refer to appropriate providers

       b.   Monitor and evaluate response to services to ensure that needs are met; emotionally, physically, and financially

  3. Clinician

       a.   Holistic practice: the developing child has a broad range of interacting needs in many settings that affect the collective health of the "client" as a larger system

       b.   Focus on wellness: promote health and prevention of illness in child and adolescent population

       c.   Expanded skills: with this population, skills are broad; safety and environmental concerns, knowledge of growth and development, anticipatory guidance, substance abuse and mental health counseling, dealing with limited funding for child health programs, collaboration with consumers, professionals, community organizations

4. Collaborator: work with consumers of health care, community members, professionals

5. Counselor: listen to individual clients, their families, to providers of services; assist them in finding internal and community resources to meet needs

6. **Educator: greatest role, in time and talent, with the child and adolescent population; through the parent, the child, or larger systems providing services to this population**

7. Researcher

   a. Consumer of research: remain up-to-date on changes in child care practice; use this information to change practice and promote quality and effectiveness

   b. Producer of research: seek opportunities to conduct research alone or in collaboration with others to enhance the knowledge base in the field of child health

IV. Adult and Work-Related Health

A. Specific Needs

1. Growth and development will proceed successfully uninterrupted by illness or injury and enhanced by the client who practices healthy living practices.

2. The adult lives and works in a safe and healthful environment; the adult assumes responsible positions demonstrated in thought and action.

3. The adult receives appropriate immunizations (adult tetanus–diptheria toxoid [Td] every 10 years), screening, and health education to promote a high level of wellness.

4. Learning and productivity are lifelong.

5. Adults are role models for youth and children.

B. Goals of Healthy People 2000: Selected Goals of Healthy People 2000 for Adults (Display 14-4)

C. Levels of Prevention

1. Primary

   a. Teach healthy living habits to keep illness or injury from ever occurring in the adult population

   b. Provide adults with anticipatory guidance to prepare them for challenges associated with changing parental and work-related responsibilities and continued aging

   c. **Provide adults with self-care skills and the assertiveness needed to be an effective health care consumer in a changing health care environment**

2. Secondary

   a. Early diagnosis and treatment: identified through screening procedures to detect, diagnose, and treat age-related health concerns (cholesterol levels, diabetes, hypertension,

DISPLAY 14-4.
Selected Goals of *Healthy People 2000* for Adults

OBJECTIVE	1987 BASELINE	2000 TARGET
Reduce the death rate for adults to no more than 340 per 100,000 people through age 64	423	340
Increase to at least 85% the proportion of women age 18 and older with uterine cervix who received a Pap test within the preceding 1 to 3 years	75	85
Reduce alcohol consumption by people age 14 and older to an annual average of no more than 2 gallons of ethanol per person	2.54	2.0
Reduce diabetes to an incidence of no more than 2.5 per 1,000 people and a prevalence of no more than 25 per 1,000 people	2.9 28	2.5 25

vision and hearing changes, STDs, abuse, violence) at the earliest possible stage to encourage a return to wellness

    b. Prompt treatment of injuries related to falls, crashes, or violence that can occur related to recreation, motor vehicles, or violence at home or in the community

  3. Tertiary

    a. Initiate rehabilitation to minimize effects on the adult; return to the highest level of wellness; in some cases to extend and save the adult's life

    b. Attempt to reduce the extent and severity of an illness; hepatitis, tuberculosis, AIDS, pneumonia, arthritis, asthma, substance use, cancer, effects of work-related exposure to toxins, depression, heart disease, osteoporosis

    c. Attempt to reduce the extent and severity of injuries; wounds, broken bones, internal injuries at home or work

D. Selected Skills of the Community Health Nurse

  1. Advocate

    a. Speak out for the clients; cut "red-tape" to receive appropriate adult health services

    b. Take broad adult health concerns to the appropriate problem solver; local, state, or federal level; speak professionally on behalf of needed changes

  2. Case manager

    a. Assess, plan, and coordinate adult health services; refer to appropriate providers

    b. Monitor and evaluate response to services to ensure that needs are met emotionally, physically, and financially

3. Clinician
   a. Holistic practice: the adult has a broad range of interacting needs in many settings and roles that affect the collective health of the "client" as a larger system
   b. Focus on wellness: promote health and prevention of illness and injury in adult populations
   c. Expanded skills: with this population, skills are broad; safety and environmental concerns, substance abuse and mental health counseling, limited funding for adult health programs, social and financial concerns, collaboration with consumers, professionals, organizations and community groups
4. Collaborator: work with consumers of health care, community members, professionals
5. Counselor: listen to individual clients, extended family members, and providers of services; assist them in finding internal and community resources to meet needs

6. **Educator: greatest role, in time and talent, with the adult population; through the individual or larger systems that provides services to this population**
7. Researcher
   a. Consumer of research: remain up-to-date on changes in adult health practice; use this information to change practice and promote quality and effectiveness
   b. Producer of research: seek opportunities to conduct research alone or in collaboration with others to enhance the knowledge base in the field of adult health

V. Older Adult Health
A. Specific Needs
   1. Growth and development will proceed successfully uninterrupted by illness or injury and enhanced by the older adult client who practices healthy living practices.
   2. The older adult lives, recreates (and may work) in a safe and healthful environment; the older adult assumes a satisfying position in the community, which is demonstrated in thought and action.
   3. The older adult receives appropriate immunizations (pneumonia, flu, adult Td), screening (TB, prostate-specific antigen [PSA], breast exams, cholesterol), and health education to promote a high level of wellness.
   4. Years of disability should be compressed so the older adult has more years of good health and optimal functioning with chronic diseases.

     5.   Learning and productivity are lifelong and should be encouraged.

     6.   Older adults are role models for adults, youth, and children.

B.   **Goals of Healthy People 2000: Selected Goals of Healthy People 2000 for Older Adults (Display 14-5)**

C.   **Levels of Prevention**

     1.   Primary

        a.   Teach healthy living habits to keep illness or injury from ever occurring in the older adult population

        b.   **Prevent falls among older adults (especially threatening to quality of life)**

        c.   Provide older adults with anticipatory guidance to prepare them for challenges associated with aging such as retirement, losses due to death, income changes, and their own mortality

        d.   **Provide older adults with self-care skills and the assertiveness needed to be an effective health care consumer in a changing health care environment and with continued changes in Medicare**

     2.   Secondary

        a.   Early diagnosis and treatment: identified through screening procedures to detect, diagnose, and treat age-related health concerns (cholesterol levels, diabetes, arthritis, hypertension, vision and hearing changes, STDs, abuse, violence) at the earliest possible stage to encourage a high level of wellness

        b.   Prompt treatment of injuries related to falls, crashes, or violence that occurs during recreation, activities of daily living, motor vehicles, or from violence at home or in the community

DISPLAY 14-5.
Selected Goals of *Healthy People 2000* for Older Adults

OBJECTIVE	1987 BASELINE	2000 TARGET
Reduce suicide among white men age 65 and older to no more than 39.2 per 100,000	46.1	39.2
Reduce deaths among people age 65 through 84 from falls and fall-related injuries to no more than 14.4 per 100,000	18	14.4
Reduce epidemic-related pneumonia and influenza deaths among people age 65 and older to no more than 7.3 per 100,000	9.1	7.3

3. Tertiary
   a. Initiate rehabilitation to minimize effects on the older adult; return to the highest level of wellness; in some cases to extend and save the older adult's life and quality of life
   b. Attempt to reduce the extent and severity of an illness; hepatitis, tuberculosis, AIDS, pneumonia, flu, arthritis, asthma, substance use, cancer, depression, heart disease, osteoporosis
   c. Attempt to reduce the extent and severity of injuries; wounds, broken bones, internal injuries at home or at leisure

D. Selected Skills of the Community Health Nurse
   1. Advocate
      a. Speak out for older adults; cut "red-tape" to receive appropriate health services for the elderly
      b. Take broad concerns to the appropriate problem solver; local, state, or federal level; speak professionally on behalf of needed changes
   2. Case manager
      a. Assess, plan, and coordinate older adult health services; refer to appropriate providers
      b. Monitor and evaluate response to services to ensure that needs are met emotionally, physically, and financially
   3. Clinician
      a. Holistic practice: the older adult has a broad range of interacting needs that increases with age and affects the collective health of the "client" as a larger system
      b. Focus on wellness: promote health and prevention of illness and injury in older adult populations
      c. Expanded skills: with this population, skills are broad; safety and environmental concerns, substance abuse and mental health counseling, dealing with limited and decreasing funding for older adult health programs, social and financial concerns, collaboration with consumers, professionals, community organizations
   4. Collaborator: work with consumers, community members, professionals to promote the health of elders
   5. Counselor: listen to individual clients, extended family members, and providers of services; assist them in finding internal and community resources to meet needs
   6. **Educator: greatest role, in time and talent, with the older adult population; individually or through larger systems providing services to this population**

 7. Researcher
  a. Consumer of research: remain up-to-date on changes in older adult health practice; use this information to change practice and promote quality and effectiveness
  b. Producer of research: seek opportunities to conduct research alone or in collaboration with others to enhance the knowledge base in the field of older adult health

Bibliography

Spradley, B. W., & Allender, J. A. (1996). *Community health nursing: Concepts and practice.* (4th ed.). Philadelphia: Lippincott-Raven.

Stanhope, M., & Lancaster, J. (1992). *Community health nursing: Process and practice for promoting Health* (3rd ed.). St. Louis: Mosby–Year Book.

Swanson, J. M., & Albrecht, M. (1993). *Community health nursing: Promoting the health of aggregates.* Philadelphia: W.B. Saunders.

US Department of Health and Human Services, Public Health Service. (1991). *Healthy people 2000: National health promotion and disease prevention objectives.* Washington, DC: US Government Printing Office.

STUDY QUESTIONS

1. Healthy People 2000 is a:
   a. New video on longevity and aging in the 21st century
   b. Program to improve the health of people in Third World countries
   c. Government document with health goals for Americans in the 1990s
   d. Way of looking at the health of people, through their own eyes

2. A specific need of the maternal-aged (15 to 45) population in the United States is:
   a. Postponing pregnancy until at least age 25
   b. If sexually active, being able to decide when pregnancy occurs
   c. Curtailing pregnancies after age 35 due to the higher risk
   d. Making sure there are available acute care facilities for delivery

3. The selected maternal and infant population objectives from Display 14-2 indicate that:
   a. Some objectives had worse statistics in 1990 than indicated in 1987 data
   b. We are making progress in reducing low birth weight babies among blacks
   c. Among the selected objectives, improvement in statistics has been rapid
   d. Cesarean delivery rates are at approximately 10% nationwide

4. An example of primary prevention with the maternal–infant population is to:
   a. Diagnose problem pregnancies early in order to begin treatment
   b. Encourage proper diet, rest, exercise, and regular prenatal care
   c. Follow health care practitioner recommendations for illness care
   d. Detecting signs and symptoms of infection and premature labor

5. An example of the advocate role of the community health nurse with the maternal–infant population includes:
   a. Assessing, planning, and coordinating maternal–infant services
   b. Listening to clients, assisting them to find resources that meet needs
   c. Teaching clients how to promote a healthy pregnancy
   d. Take broad concerns to the appropriate person to solve problems

6. Selected Healthy People 2000 objectives among the child-aged population include:
   a. Reduce the death rate of children to no more than 28 per 100,000 children
   b. Reduce cigarette smoking to no more that 30% in youth under age 20
   c. Enact handgun laws protecting children, in at least half of the states
   d. Childhood deaths from motor vehicle crashes lowered to less than 10 per 100,000

7. Selected goals for adults in Healthy People 2000 include:
   a. Decrease the death rate for adults to 200 per 100,000
   b. Increase the percentage of women who have Pap tests to at least 50%
   c. Reduce alcohol consumption to no more than 4 gallons of ethanol per person
   d. Reduce diabetes incidence to no more than 2.5 per 1,000 people

8. An example of secondary prevention with the adult population includes:
   a. Early diagnosis and treatment of chronic illnesses, such as diabetes
   b. Teaching healthy living habits to keep illnesses from occurring
   c. Provide adults with self-care skills to be an effective health care consumer
   d. Attempt to reduce the extent and severity of injuries that have occurred

9. Selected goals of Healthy People 2000 for older adults include reducing:
   a. Suicides among older white men to no more than 50 per 100,000

b. Deaths from falls and fall-related injuries to no more than 25 per 100,000

c. Epidemic pneumonia and flu deaths to no more than 7.3 per 100,000

d. The percentage of older adults in the US population

10. The case manager role of the community health nurse with older adults includes:

a. Monitoring and evaluating the responses of older adults to provided services

b. Speaking out for older adults, making it easier for them to receive quality care

c. Focusing on wellness when providing care to older adults

d. Working cooperatively with others to promote the health of elders

ANSWER KEY

1. *Correct response: c*
Answer choices **a, b,** and **d** are incorrect responses.
Comprehension/Safe Care/Assessment

2. *Correct response: b*
Answer choices **a** and **c** suggest specific ages for pregnancy and are inappropriate. Individuals are different, and no one age is right for all people. Answer choice **d** implies there are inadequate facilities for infant delivery. This is not a major problem in the United States. Most people live within reasonable distances from facilities with maternity services.
Application/Safe Care/Planning

3. *Correct response: a*
The birth weight statistics for black infants in 1990 were worse than in 1987, making answer choice **b** incorrect.
Answer choice **c** suggests the statistics have improved in all of the selected areas. This in incorrect.
Cesarean delivery rates are over 24% nationwide, making answer choice **d** incorrect.
Analysis/Health Promotion/Evaluation

4. *Correct response: b*
Answers **a** and **c** are examples of secondary prevention, and answer choice **d** is an example of tertiary prevention.
Application/Safe Care/Implementation

5. *Correct response: d*
Answers **a, b,** and **c** are examples of case manager, educator, and counselor roles, respectively.
Application/Health Promotion/Implementation

6. *Correct response: a*
Answer choice **b** is 15%; answer choice **c**—the objective expects the state law to change in all 50 states; and in choice **d**—5.5 % is the goal.
Comprehension/Safe Care/Analysis

7. *Correct choice: d*
Answer choice **a** is 340 people per 100,000; **b** is 85% of women; **c** is 2 gallons of ethanol.
Application/Health Promotion/Implementation

8. *Correct choice: a*
Answer choices **b** and **c** are examples of secondary prevention.
Answer choice **d** is an example of tertiary prevention.
Application/Health Promotion/Implementation

9. *Correct choice: c*
In answer choice **a**, the number is 39.2 per 100,000.
Choice **b** is 14.4 per 100,000.
Answer choice **d** is incorrect because there is no attempt to reduce the numbers of older adults. The numbers are increasing from the present 12% to over 20% by the year 2030.
Application/Health Promotion/Implementation

10. *Correct response: a*
Answer choice **b** is an example of the advocate role.
Choice **c** is an example of the clinician role.
Choice **d** is an example of the collaborator role.
Application/Health Promotion/Implementation

Health Care Needs
of a Stressed Society

I.   Poverty
A.   Levels of Prevention

1.   Primary: basic education; adult education; job training, employment; positive mental health practices; access to positive role models; strong family support systems; accessible medical, mental health, and social services

2. Secondary: empowerment; advocacy; assistance in getting immediate needs met; short- and long-term planning; retraining
3. Tertiary: access to positive role models; comprehensive social services; long-term planning; innovative programs led by community members; medical and mental health services; retraining programs

B. Societal Issues

1. Morbidity and mortality rates are higher among people in poverty.
2. Deprivation is associated with:
    a. Poor nutrition: affects well-being, causes illnesses
    b. Inferior and overcrowded living conditions: increases illnesses
    c. Less than optimal lifestyle behaviors: causes frustration leading to emotional or physical abuse (substance abuse, gang membership)

    d. **Uninsured and underinsured health care: limits use of and access to health services; primary prevention is not a priority—survival is a priority; emergency room is used as primary entry into the health care system**
    e. Inadequate educational levels: low wages; reliance on federal assistance programs; low self-esteem; powerlessness; hopelessness; helplessness
    f. Low wages: limits options and buying power
    g. Crime: a means to have what others have; to acquire drugs; express anger and frustration; become accepted; enter gangs
    h. Gangs: means of survival, acceptance, belonging

3. **People raised in poverty tend to stay in poverty, perpetuating the problem.**

C. Specific Services

1. These innovative programs are holistic in nature.
2. The programs are designed to empower the individual.
3. The programs focus on:
    a. Educational experiences that are culturally relevant
    b. Employment training
    c. Accessible health care services
    d. Recreational and social services that promote independence from public assistance

II. Homelessness

A. Levels of Prevention

1. Primary: education; training, employment; regular savings plan; living within one's means; positive mental health prac-

tices; develop wide support systems among family members, friends, religious organizations

2. Secondary: safe shelters; assistance with immediate needs; innovative programs to keep families together and reestablish lives; adult education; retraining; medical, mental health, and social services as needed

3. Tertiary: social services; self-help programs; guidance and counseling; medical and mental health services; retraining programs; life skills classes to teach primary prevention practices

B. Societal Issues (Ugarriza & Fallon, 1994)
   1. 31% of the homeless are women.
   2. 25% of homeless women are single and have children.
   3. 30% to 40% of the homeless are mentally ill.

   4. An increasing number of the homeless are families.

C. Specific Services
   1. These innovative prevention programs are holistic in nature.
   2. The programs are designed to empower the individual
   3. The program focus on:
      a. Primary prevention through employers, creditors, accessing mental health services
      b. Educational opportunities
      c. Employment training
      d. Accessible comprehensive health care services

III. Teenage Pregnancy
   A. Levels of Prevention
      1. Primary: sex education that includes abstinence and responsible sexual behavior; accessibility to health and family planning services; supportive family systems; a rich family and school environment that includes goal setting for future education and career
      2. Secondary: prenatal care; involve the teen father; supportive family and friends; continuation with educational program; parenting classes; guidance and counseling services; alternatives to parenting, including abortion and adoption
      3. Tertiary: assistance with parenting responsibilities; child care as parent(s) finish their education; social services; counseling; medical and mental health; affordable day care after education completed so parents or mother may work

   B. Societal Issues (US Department of Commerce, 1993)
      1. 20% of all births are to adolescent females.
      2. Each year, 10% of all teenage girls become pregnant.
      3. One third of teenage pregnancies end in abortion.
      4. Babies born to teenage mothers are more likely to be premature and underweight.

5. Educational programs are interrupted or discontinued; parents having less than a high school education often become eligible for federal and state assistance.

C. Specific Services

1. Sex education is taught at home, in religious centers, at school.
2. Supportive programs are offered for pregnant teens to promote a healthy pregnancy, ensure an uneventful delivery experience, and teach parenting skills.
3. Supportive programs are offered for teen parents so education and work can continue while they provide for the young family.
4. Health care services are made physically and financially accessible, focusing on primary prevention, especially of STDs and unplanned pregnancies.

IV. Substance Abuse

A. Levels of Prevention

1. Primary: education; positive coping mechanisms; positive role models; open communication system among family members, friends, religious organizations
2. Secondary: early recognition of abuse; surveillance systems; drug testing; employee assistance; initiation of aggressive treatment; medical, mental health, and social services provided through innovative programs that work with the entire family
3. Tertiary: long-term follow-up; medical and mental health services; develop new friends and interests

B. Societal Issues

1. Commonly abused substances include alcohol, marijuana, cocaine, crack, caffeine, and tobacco.
2. More than 13 million people in the United States are dependent on or abuse alcohol (Grant et al, 1991).

n   **The World Health Organization predicts that alcoholism is becoming the world's leading health problem. Programs such as Drug Abuse Warning Network (DAWN) are being initiated.**

3. Drug dependency is an increasing societal problem and is characterized by "underachievement, loneliness, mistrust and fear of closeness, identity problems, social conflicts, and self-destructive tendencies" (Pickett & Hanlon, 1990).
4. The availability of prescription and illegal drugs promotes use.
5. The effects on society include family disruption; family neglect and abuse; increased community violence; homicide;

crime; expensive treatment and rehabilitation—often repeated and/or ineffective contributing to continuing dysfunction.

C.   **Specific Services**

   1.   Schools: educate about drugs and their dangers, include children of all ages; educate parents; educate the lay public about dependence on "safe" drugs like prescriptions, caffeine, diet pills; initiate effective drug prevention programs

   2.   Accessible diagnostic services, drug testing programs

   3.   Detoxification centers; halfway houses; support groups, like Alcoholics Anonymous (AA), Narcotics Anonymous (NA); methadone clinics

V.   Mental Illness (Display 15-1)

   A.   **Levels of Prevention**

   1.   Primary: education; teaching positive coping skills individually or in groups; positive role models; open communication systems among family members, friends, religious organizations; balance in life; stress reduction

   2.   Secondary: early recognition of signs and symptoms of illness; surveillance; initiation of treatment including medical and social services provided through innovative programs that include the entire family

   3.   Tertiary: long-term outpatient follow-up; group and individual counseling; provide alternative housing and work opportunities

DISPLAY 15-1.
Categories of Mental Disorders

- Disorders usually first evident in infancy, childhood, or adolescence
- Dissociative disorders
- Sexual disorders
- Organic mental syndromes and disorders
- Psychotic disorders not elsewhere classified
- Psychoactive substance use disorders
- Schizophrenia
- Delusional disorders
- Mood disorders
- Anxiety disorders
- Somatoform disorders
- Sleep disorders
- Factitious disorders
- Impulse control disorders not elsewhere classified
- Adjustment disorders
- Psychological factors affecting physical condition
- Personality disorders
- Conditions not attributable to a mental disorder that are a focus of attention or treatment

(In Pickett & Hanlon, 1990, from the American Psychiatric Association's Diagnostic and Statistical Manual of Mental Disorders, 1987)

B.   Societal Issues
1.   Over 224,000 mentally ill and impaired patients are being treated as inpatients (Manderscheid & Barrett, 1987).
2.   300,000 mentally ill are in nursing homes (Kiesler & Sibulkin, 1987).
3.   Numerous others remain untreated in the community, many of whom are homeless.
4.   The mentally ill have physical, emotional, and social problems that have an impact on families and communities, both emotionally and financially.

C.   Specific Services
1.   Primary: support groups; self-help groups; assertiveness training; counseling services; community health nursing
2.   Secondary: early diagnosis and treatment; definitive mental health services; drug rehabilitation
3.   Tertiary: long-term mental health follow-up; group homes; halfway houses; sheltered workshops

VI.   Developmental and Physical Challenges

A.   Levels of Prevention
1.   Primary: education about causes of developmental disabilities; abstain from drugs and alcohol during pregnancy; avoid exposure to toxic substances and exposure to infectious processes; early and regular prenatal care; prevention of accidents in children and adults; safety practices including: wearing helmets when bicycle riding and skateboarding; motor vehicle safety, which includes safe speeds, proper use of car seats, seat belts, air bags; eliminate exposure to lead; work and leisure safety practices
2.   Secondary: early recognition of signs and symptoms of a developmental disability, in utero, at birth, or after an injury or toxic exposure; surveillance; initiation of treatment including medical, physical, speech and occupational therapy and social services through innovative programs that include the whole family
3.   Tertiary: long-term inpatient, rehabilitative, and outpatient follow-up; inclusive or alternative educational programs; assistive devices; modified housing and work opportunities

B.   Societal Issues
1.   Technological advances allow preterm infants, born before 37 weeks gestation (some as early as 20 weeks' gestation), and very low birth weight babies (some weighing less than 500 grams at birth) to survive infancy.
2.   Injury, infection, and exposure to toxins rob a healthy child or adult of unlimited potential and may delay, interrupt, or halt intellectual, emotional, and physical development or ability.

    3. Some developmentally or physically disabled people are totally dependent on others to meet basic activities of daily living. This can cause stress in families and be resource intensive to communities.

C. **Specific Services**

    1. Primary: prenatal services; safe water supply; an environment free of toxins including lead, pesticides, mercury, nuclear wastes; immunization programs for children and adults; safety-related legislation; the manufacture of safe vehicles and toys

    2. Secondary: counseling services; case management; public health nursing services; innovative programs that provide aggressive rehabilitation and education

    3. Tertiary: long-term rehabilitative follow-up including counseling and therapy; group homes; sheltered workshops; modified housing options and income assistance

D. **The Nurse's Role**

    1. Educator: determine specific needs of individuals; teach basic health promotion skills

    2. Clinician: use assessment and caregiving skills to meet identified needs of individuals, families, and aggregates

    3. Advocate: assist clients in receiving services that will promote their quality of life and provide stability; interact with community resources on behalf of the client

    4. Counselor: allow clients to verbalize concerns; work with them in ways that empower and promote independence

    5. Leader: coordinate agency services with community services; plan, organize, and manage programs to promote community health and safety

    6. Researcher: use data in the literature to enhance services; participate in research that leads to effective programs on behalf of specific aggregates

VII. Violence

A. **Types of Violence**

    1. Random violence: affects the innocent, is directed toward a person or persons unknown to the attacker, is unpredictable; includes drive-by shootings, car jackings, vandalism, robbery, muggings, rape; all people are at risk

    2. Terrorism: directed toward individuals or groups, usually unknown to the terrorist, committed as an aggressive act in support of a particular political or religious ideology, as a way of sending a message to others; actions include bombings, kidnapping; hostages

    3. Gangs: a nontraditional family form in which groups of young men and women bond and substitute the gang for biologic family; gang lifestyle is counter-cultural, involves drugs

and violence toward other gang members; frequently violence involves non-gang members as the innocent are assaulted for cash and valuables; gang members gain status by committing violent acts, even killing individuals

B. Levels of Prevention

1. Primary: safety practices among individuals, groups, and at varying degrees in public places, such as airports and court houses; home safety and security; pedestrian safety, especially at night and in unfamiliar neighborhoods; parents need to know their child's friends and whereabouts at all times

2. Secondary: early detection that violence may erupt or is erupting; notify proper authorities; get to safety; first-aid; definitive medical care; counseling; support groups

3. Tertiary: reconstruct lives and communities, support families through the grieving process; rehabilitative services for victims and families; long-term follow-up

C. Societal Issues

1. Homicide from firearms is ten times more prevalent among black 15- to 19-year-old youth than white youth. It is the leading cause of death for black males in this age group (US Department of Commerce, 1993).

2. The frequency of criminal activity in some communities makes it unsafe for children to play outside or go to school.

3. Fighting crime is a major problem in the United States because it consumes resources that could be used for more productive endeavors, such as education, the arts, and recreation.

D. Specific Services

1. Primary: stranger awareness and safe home programs, activating the 911 system; neighborhood watch programs; self-defense training; support of the police force; neighborhood clean-up programs

2. Secondary: emergency response teams; definitive medical care; clergy and counseling services

3. Tertiary: long-term follow-up; self-help groups; stricter laws affecting offenders; innovative programs for gang members wanting to change their lifestyle; neighborhood reclamation programs; support federal, and cooperate with international, attempts to reduce terrorism

VIII. Abuse (Display 15-2)

A. Domestic Abuse: physical or emotional mistreatment of one's partner, which can be triggered by numerous factors, such as job loss, pregnancy, role changes, alcohol and drug abuse, childhood history of abuse and/or parental violence, mental or physical disorders

1. Primary prevention: intact self-esteem, assertiveness, healthy family life, counseling, education, anticipatory guidance

DISPLAY 15-2.
Violence in the Home—Facts about Domestic Violence

> ► One and a half million children are reported as abused or neglected each year in the United States (Straus & Gelles, 1990)
> ► Two thirds of abused children are being parented by a battered woman
> ► 25% of the world's women are violently abused in their own homes (UNICEF, 1995)
> ► Domestic violence in the United States is the largest single cause of injury to women, leading to more hospital admissions than muggings, rapes, and auto crashes combined (UNICEF, 1995)
> ► There are 32 cases of elder abuse per 1000 elderly persons in the United States each year (Hyde-Robertson, Pirnie, & Freeze, 1994)

2. Secondary prevention: police intervention, first-aid, definitive medical treatment, battered women's shelter (temporary safety from another violent episode), counseling
3. Tertiary prevention: court protective orders, restraining orders, counseling, moving away to permanent safety, personal development courses, which include self-esteem building and assertiveness

B. Child Abuse: maltreatment of children including any or all of the following: physical, emotional, medical, or educational neglect; physical, emotional or sexual maltreatment and exploitation (Spradley & Allender, 1996) (Display 15-3).

1. Primary prevention: perinatal programs, healthy family life practices, effective parenting skills, support groups, respite programs, parental stress hotlines, family assessment for high-risk behaviors

DISPLAY 15-3.
Mandated Reporting of Abuse

Mandated Reporter

In most states, certain professionals who work with children such as day care providers, teachers, nurses, social workers, and doctors are required by law to report suspected child abuse and are breaking a state law if they do not report suspected abuse.

Community health nurses are mandated reporters.

California Child Abuse and Neglect (Crime Prevention Center, 1993)

The Mandated Reporter Law in California includes child care custodians, health practitioners, child protective agency staff, and commercial film and photographic print processors. A professional who fails to make a required report is guilty of a misdemeanor punishable by up to 6 months in jail and/or up to a $1000 fine.

A required report must be initiated immediately (or as soon as practically possible) by phone and followed within 36 hours by a written report submitted to a child protective agency on Department of Justice forms.

    2. Secondary prevention: early recognition and intervention; reporting required by law if child abuse is suspected by nurses, physicians, or other professionals who work with children; medical and emotional care; law enforcement; protective services and foster care

    3. Tertiary prevention: long-term follow-up, which includes family counseling and reunification activities, short- or long-term foster care, medical rehabilitation, personal counseling

C. **Elder Abuse: mistreatment of elders falls into two categories: abuse—physical, psychological, financial, and sexual; neglect—active and passive**

    1. Primary prevention: healthy family life practices; effective caregiving plans; preparedness for caregiving costs; support groups; respite programs; caregiver stress hotlines; in-service education for long-term care staff

    2. Secondary prevention: early recognition and intervention, medical and emotional care, adult protective services, law enforcement

    3. Tertiary prevention: long-term follow-up, which includes family counseling, medical rehabilitation, personal counseling, placement or relocation services

D. **The Nurse's Responsibilities**

    1. Reporting: In most states, the community health nurse is designated as a mandated reporter, and suspected abuse must be reported.

    2. Collaborating: Effective resolution of abusive situations require interprofessional collaboration among staff in appropriate agencies.

    3. Follow-up: The community health nurse frequently stays involved with the family and provides needed support, such as health assessment, education, and referrals.

IX. **Disasters**

  A. **Definitions**

    1. Disaster: any occurrence, natural or manmade, that interrupts the normal day-to-day life of individuals, groups, or communities

      a. Natural: disasters related to phenomena occurring in nature, such as tornados, hurricanes, monsoons, floods, earthquakes, lightening strike fires, volcanic eruptions, land slides, blizzards

      b. Manmade: disasters that occur related to manmade phenomena, such as transportation crashes, terrorist bombings, wars, fires, oil rig and mining deaths, nuclear accidents, exposure to toxic substances

B. Levels of Prevention

1. Primary: knowledge of risk factors, individual and community preparedness, safety practices
2. Secondary: immediate rescue, prevention of additional injury or death after the initial occurrence, first-aid, organized community response, definitive medical care, shelters, family location and identification services
3. Tertiary: long-term alternative shelter, relocation services, family and community rehabilitation

C. Societal Issues

1. Physical: loss of life, limb, and property
2. Emotional: disruption in family, group, and community functioning; long-lasting emotional effects
3. Financial cost: to individuals, groups and communities may be massive; undermines the economy of a region, state, or the country

D. Specific Services

1. The American Red Cross (ARC): a quasi-official agency; federally mandated to provide community disaster services through shelters, first-aid, air-flight teams, and assistance to those in the military at no cost to the individual; local chapters may provide multiple other services, such as blood banking; CPR, first-aid, and teen babysitting classes
2. The Federal Emergency Management Agency (FEMA): provides low-interest loans to individuals, groups, and communities to reconstruct lost homes and businesses in federally declared disaster areas
3. Public health services: water testing for purity, mass immunizations to prevent infectious diseases; educating the public; home visits; case management

E. The Nurse's Role

1. Educator: teach individuals about preparedness, especially in communities prone to specific disasters
2. Clinician: coordinate agency services with ARC in your community; volunteer as a shelter nurse with ARC
3. Advocate: assist families affected by the disaster to achieve stability; speak for them; acquire needed services and supplies
4. Counselor: allow client to verbalize fears and feelings; assist with working through losses and the grieving process; provide guidance to restore "normalcy" to lives
5. Leader: plan, organize, and manage programs to promote community health and safety

Bibliography

Crime Prevention Center. (1993). *Child abuse prevention handbook.* Sacramento, CA: Office of the Attorney General.

Grant, B. F., Harford, T., Chou, P., et al. (1991). Prevalence of SDM-III-R alcohol abuse and dependence: United States, 1988. *Alcohol Health Research World, 15,* 91–96.

Hyde-Robertson, B., Pirnie, S. M., & Freeze, C. (1994). A strategy against elderly mistreatment. *CARING Magazine, 11,* 40–44.

Kiesler, C. A., & Sibulkin, A. E. (1987). *Mental hospitalization: Myths and facts about a national crisis.* Newbury Park, CA: Sage.

Manderscheid, R. W., & Barrett, S. A. (Eds.). (1987). *Mental health, U.S. 1987.* Rockville, MD: US Department of Health and Human Services.

Pickett, G., & Hanlon, J. (1990). *Public health: Administration and practice* (9th ed.). St. Louis: Times Mirror/Mosby.

Spradley, B. W., & Allender, J. A. (1996). *Community health nursing: Concepts and practice.* (4th ed.). Philadelphia: Lippincott-Raven.

Stanhope, M., & Lancaster, J. (1992). *Community health nursing: Process and practice for promoting health* (3rd ed.). St. Louis: Mosby–Year Book.

Straus, M. A., & Gelles, R. J. (1990). *Physical violence in American families: Risk factors and adaptions to violence in 8,145 families.* New Brunswick, NJ: Transaction.

Ugarriza, D. N., & Fallon, T. (1994). Nurse's attitudes toward homeless women: A barrier to change. *Nursing Outlook, 42*(1), 26–29.

UNICEF. (1995). *The state of the world's children 1995.* New York: Oxford.

US Department of Commerce. (1993). *US statistical abstracts* (113th ed.). Washington, DC: Author.

STUDY QUESTIONS

1. Populations in poverty experience higher rates of:
   a. Mortality
   b. Employment
   c. Mental health
   d. Education

2. Homelessness is an increasing problem in the United States. Which of the following groups of homeless is increasing?
   a. Older men
   b. Families
   c. Teenagers
   d. Mentally ill

3. An example of primary prevention of teenage pregnancy includes:
   a. Adoption
   b. Abortion
   c. Sex education
   d. Prenatal care

4. Teenage pregnancy remains a societal issue in that:
   a. Each year 10% of teenage girls become pregnant
   b. 10% of all births are to adolescent females
   c. Half of teenage pregnancies end in abortion
   d. Pregnant teens finish high school but do not go on to college

5. Substance abuse in the United States is characterized by:
   a. 5 million people dependent on or abusing alcohol
   b. Difficulty in accessing prescription and illegal drugs
   c. Inexpensive and successful rehabilitation programs
   d. Increased family disruption, violence, and crime

6. An example of secondary prevention when working with the mentally ill population includes:
   a. Long-term follow-up
   b. Sheltered workshops
   c. Definitive mental health services
   d. Alternative housing arrangements

7. Preventing developmental and physical disabilities at the primary level includes the following activities:
   a. Early recognition of the signs and symptoms of illness
   b. Abstaining from drugs and alcohol during pregnancy
   c. Inpatient, rehabilitative, and outpatient follow-up
   d. Initiating treatment through innovative programs

8. Violence directed toward individuals or groups, committed as an aggressive act in support of a particular political or religious ideology is characteristic of:
   a. Gang activity
   b. Random violence
   c. Terrorist behavior
   d. Domestic violence

9. Facts about violence in the home include:
   a. 500,000 children are reported as abused or neglected each year
   b. Domestic violence is a problem in the United States, but practically unheard of in other countries
   c. Elder abuse is rare with less than 2 cases per 1000 older adults
   d. Domestic violence is the largest single cause of injury to women requiring hospitalization

10. A community health nurse responds to a part of town affected by a flooding river due to heavy rains and administers immunizations because the public water supply is contaminated and waterborne disease may occur. This is an example of what type of disaster, what level of disaster prevention, and what level of illness prevention?
    a. Manmade disaster; primary disaster prevention; secondary illness prevention
    b. Natural disaster; secondary disaster prevention; primary illness prevention

c. Natural disaster; primary disaster prevention; primary illness prevention

d. Manmade disaster; tertiary disaster prevention; secondary illness prevention

ANSWER KEY

1. *Correct response: a*
The population in poverty has higher rates of unemployment, mental illness, and less education.
Comprehension/NA/Assessment

2. *Correct response: b*
Other groups are homeless in great numbers, but families were not a traditional homeless population and their numbers are increasing.
Comprehension/NA/Assessment

3. *Correct response: c*
Answer choices **a, b,** and **d** are examples of secondary prevention.
Application/Health Promotion/ Implementation

4. *Correct response: a*
Answer choice **b** is incorrect. The percentage is 20%.
Answer choice **c** is higher than the one third that ends in abortion.
Answer choice **d** is incorrect. Pregnancy disrupts school, and many teens discontinue their high school education.
Comprehension/NA/Assessment

5. *Correct response: d*
Answer choice **a** is incorrect. The number is 13 million.
Answer choice **b** is incorrect. Unfortunately, prescription and illegal drugs are readily available.
Answer choice **c**—rehabilitative programs are expensive and the programs are often unsuccessful and repeated, which is a major problem.
Comprehension/Health Promotion/ Analysis

6. *Correct response: c*
Answer choices **a, b,** and **d** are examples of tertiary prevention services.
Application/Health Promotion/ Implementation

7. *Correct response: b*
Answer choices **a** and **d** are examples of tertiary prevention. Answer choice **c** is an example of secondary prevention.
Application/Health Promotion/ Implementation

8. *Correct response: c*
Answer choices **a, b,** and **d** describe other categories of violence present in society.
Comprehension/Psychosocial/Analysis

9. *Correct response: d*
Answer choice **a** is a low number. 1.5 million children are reported as abused or neglected each year in the Unites States.
Answer choice **b**—25% of the world's women are violently abused in their own homes. It is a worldwide problem.
Answer choice **c** underestimates the problem of elder abuse; 32 of 1000 elders are reported abused in the United States each year.
Comprehension/Psychosocial/Analysis

10. *Correct response: b*
This is a natural disaster, a natural phenomenon. The community health nurse is attempting to eliminate an additional problem caused by the flood by immunizing the vulnerable community members, a goal in secondary prevention during a disaster. By immunizing populations, the illness prevention is at the primary level.
Analysis/Safe Care/Implementation

Communicable Diseases:
Prevention and Control

I. Communicable Disease Control

A. Definitions

 1. Epidemiologic terminology, frequency rates, and models assist in understanding disease processes. These are basic to prevention, surveillance, and control of disease and are foundational to communicable disease control. (See Chap. 7.)

2. *Vector:* nonhuman agent that actively carries disease organisms to humans, such as insects and rodents

3. *Reservoir:* person, animal, insect, or inanimate material in which an infectious agent lives and multiplies, and which can be a source of infection to others (Spradley & Allender, 1996)

4. *Incubation period:* time interval between exposure and onset of symptoms

5. *Vaccine:* preparation made either from killed, living, attenuated, or living fully virulent organisms, introduced into the body to produce or artificially increase immunity to a specific disease by causing the formation of antibodies (Spradley & Allender, 1996)

6. *Immunization:* process of protecting an individual from a disease through introduction of a live, killed, or partial component of the invading organism into the individual's system (Stanhope & Lancaster, 1992)
7. *Surveillance:* monitoring process used to detect all aspects of communicable disease occurrence

B. Barriers

1. Medical: disease organisms mutate or change over time. This is due to inappropriate medication regimens related to client non-compliance or variations in provider treatment schedules. This causes diseases that:
    a. Are difficult to diagnose
    b. Present different or subacute symptoms
    c. Are resistant to standard treatment
2. Social: low educational levels; lack of knowledge about the effects of certain practices; value system differences; families on limited incomes with more immediate needs; transportation difficulties; time-consuming and intellectually challenging immunization paperwork; provider availability and requirements for care
3. Cultural: language barriers; differing concepts of health care and preventive measures; traditional beliefs that are in conflict with the community standard
4. Religious: some groups object to immunizations on religious grounds; courts support sincere objectors; problems arise when exempt groups live in one community or attend the same school creating a large pool of underimmunized people
5. Provider: may cause a barrier by:
    a. "Missed opportunities": overlooking an opportunity to immunize when a child comes for care for a different reason
    b. Erroneously refusing to immunize because of a mild illness that does not interfere with the immunization
    c. Erroneously refusing to administer all immunizations for which the child is due
    d. Not having the resources to keep track or to notify parents of routine immunization times
    e. Not encouraging clients to maintain their own records of immunizations

C. Responsibilities of the Community Health Nurse

1. Know the signs and symptoms of common and emerging communicable diseases.
2. Teach communicable disease control measures to at-risk populations.
3. Provide immunization programs that meet the needs of the community (assess, plan, publicize, implement, evaluate).

4. Ensure that an accurate record-keeping system of communicable disease occurrence and immunizations is in place.
5. Teach and reinforce appropriate treatment regimens when communicable diseases occur.
6. Assist in reducing or eliminating client and provider barriers to acquiring immunizations.

D. Levels of Prevention
1. Primary
   a. Community education
   b. Immunizations
2. Secondary
   a. Screening for disease
   b. Early diagnosis and treatment
3. Tertiary
   a. Isolation and quarantine
   b. Safe handling of infectious waste
   c. Preventing transmission by health care worker practices

II. Specific Communicable Diseases (Table 16-1)
A. Food and Waterborne Diseases
1. Food and waterborne diseases found in the United States include:
   a. Bacterial contamination (*Salmonella, Shigella, Escherichia coli, Staphylococcus aureus, Clostridium perfringens*)
   b. Viral contamination (hepatitis A)
   c. Protozoan contamination (*Giardia lamblia*)
2. Onset and symptoms
   a. Onset: within a few hours, days, or weeks after exposure, depending on the organism

TABLE 16-1.
Cases of Specific Notifiable Communicable Diseases—1995

DISEASE	NUMBER OF CASES	DISEASE	NUMBER OF CASES
AIDS	71,547	Syphilis (primary and secondary)	16,500
Botulism	97	Tetanus	41
Brucellosis	98	Toxic shock syndrome	191
Chlamydia	477,638	Trichinosis	29
Cholera	23	Tuberculosis	22,860
Gonorrhea	392,848	Typhoid fever	369
Lyme disease	11,700	Varicella	120,624
Measles	309		
Plague	9		

From Centers for Disease Control and Prevention. (1996). Morbidity and Mortality Weekly Report, 44 (No. 53).

        b.   Symptoms: diarrhea, nausea, vomiting, stomach cramps, jaundice

    3.   Levels of prevention

        a.   Primary: teach basic methods for preventing food and water contamination at all levels (eg, public water supply, meat-processing plants, commercial food handling and at home) (Display 16-1)

        b.   Secondary: support early diagnosis of the disease and initiation of symptom-related treatment; reinforce compliance to treatment regimen

        c.   Tertiary: support care of client; epidemiologic follow-up; interrupt and eliminate cause at the source

B. **Vector-borne Diseases**

    1.   Vector-borne diseases found in the United States include diseases caused by:

        a.   Ticks (Lyme disease, tick typhus, relapsing fever)

        b.   Fleas (plague, typhus)

        c.   Domestic and wild animals (rabies)

        d.   Mosquitos (malaria)

        e.   Louse-borne diseases (typhus, relapsing fever)

    2.   Levels of prevention

        a.   Primary: teach basic methods for preventing vector-borne diseases; teach clients to reduce insect vectors by eliminating insect-breeding areas; use mosquito netting, screens, protective clothing, insect and flea sprays; reduce population of other animal hosts that harbor the vector (rat extermination eliminates the risk of plague); teach actions to take when exposed to a vector to prevent diseases from developing or to receive prompt treatment

        b.   Secondary: support early diagnosis of the disease and initiate symptom-related treatment; reinforce compliance to treatment regimen during home visits or when in clinic

DISPLAY 16-1.
Safe Handling of Food

1. Before handling food—wash hands, wash all food preparation surfaces and utensils.
2. When preparing food—use clean water and wash food that will be eaten raw and uncooked.
3. Cook all meat products thoroughly—meat and meat juices should not be red or pink.
4. Do not allow cooked foods to come in contact with dishes or utensils used for raw meats without thorough cleaning.
5. Storing foods—cool cooked foods quickly by placing in clean covered containers; store in a refrigerator below 40°F; do not let food sit out—picnic foods should be served quickly and kept covered while serving, kept in a cooler when not serving.
6. Reheating foods—heat foods thoroughly to above 140°F.

  c. Tertiary: support care of client with epidemiologic follow-up; work with interprofessional team members (environmentalists, laboratory personnel) to interrupt or eliminate the problem

C. **Sexually Transmitted Diseases (STDS)**

  1. Common sexually transmitted diseases found in the United States include:

   a. Syphilis: caused by a spirochete—*Treponema pallidum;* enters through the bloodstream; symptoms are subtle and often missed; a highly infectious chancre (a painless sore where the organism entered the body), a generalized rash (with hallmark rash on palms and soles of the feet), followed by unpredictable, severe, systemic involvement with disability or death; disease responds well to antibiotic therapy in the primary, secondary, and early latent stage

   b. **Gonorrhea: a sexually transmitted bacterial disease caused by *Neisseria gonorrhoeae;* high-risk groups include African Americans, adolescents, and women of childbearing age; presents as a drainage from the penis or vagina, usually very noticeable in males and absent in females; progression of untreated disease leads to serious reproductive system involvement and subsequent infertility; the fetus of an untreated woman can be infected, causing complications, which could lead to death**

   c. Chlamydia: the most common sexually transmitted bacterial infection in the United States; nearly 5 million acute infections annually; case report is required in most states in the United States; can cause pelvic inflammatory disease (PID) leading to infertility in women; leads to epididymitis and infertility in men, and infant conjunctivitis and pneumonia in children

   d. Genital herpes and genital warts: annual incidence—200,000 cases/year with prevalence estimates of genital herpes infection as high as 30 million; control is difficult, many infected are asymptomatic; there is no cure; recurrent episodes may be relieved with short-term courses of acyclovir; long-term course of suppressive therapy may reduce frequency of recurrences; genital warts caused by some types of human papillomavirus (HPV) are closely associated with cervical dysplasia and genital cancers; 5% of all STD clinic visits are for genital HPV infections; infection can be passed to newborns during vaginal delivery

  2. Levels of prevention

   a. Primary: STD prevention information in the curricula of middle, junior high and high schools; innovative and effective sexual health promotion approaches in schools; act as a resource to schools, school health personnel and to staff in other settings such as in youth organizations

    b.   Secondary: increase the number of clinics offering STD screening, diagnosis, treatment, counseling and referral services; improve access to comprehensive services; case management needs to conform to CDC recommendations of medical treatment, follow-up strategies that ensure cure (if possible), notification and treatment of sexual partners

    c.   Tertiary: expanded contact tracing efforts; rehabilitative and reconstructive care to promote the highest possible quality of life

D. HIV/AIDS

    1.   History and facts

        a.   A retrovirus that attacks the body's immune system

        b.   First recognized as a distinct syndrome in 1981

        c.   Transmitted from person to person through vaginal and penile secretions during sexual contact; sharing HIV-contaminated intravenous needles and syringes; through transfusion of infected blood or its components

    2.   Treatments and prevention

        a.   No known cure; multidrug treatment regimens prolong life and improve the quality of life; people living with AIDS (PLWA) are becoming a new group now considered chronically ill; many people are living 10 to 12 years after initial diagnosis; case-fatality rate nears 100%; victims succumb to opportunistic diseases, such as pneumocystic pneumonia, tuberculosis (TB), cancer; recent medication regimens are improving the quality of life and prolonging life

        b.   **Primary prevention is vital: safe sex; elimination of sharing needles and syringes among IV drug users; safe blood and blood products supply (the blood supply in the United States has been considered safe since 1987); health care workers and others must use standard precautions**

E. Tuberculosis

    1.   History and facts

        a.   1900s and earlier called "consumption"; the disease appeared to consume victims with weight loss and eventual death

        b.   Was once nearly eradicated, now poses a major threat to the health of most nations

        c.   Current trends in the United States include sharp disparate rates among minority populations (especially immigrants and refugees); fatal association with HIV infection and AIDS; increasing rates among children; proliferation of multidrug-resistant strains

 d. **Kills 3 million people worldwide each year, more than any other single infectious disease, despite the availability of effective antituberculosis drugs since the 1940s**

 e. **In recent history, TB has been rarely treated in acute care settings in the United States; many young physicians and hospital-based nurses are unfamiliar with the disease unless associated with HIV/AIDS; TB symptomology is very subtle early in the disease; most classification III clients are physically able and not infectious after 2 weeks of drug therapy and are treated in the community**

2. Causative factors, symptoms, diagnosis, and treatment
   a. Causative organism: *Mycobacterium tuberculosis* is inhaled through airborne droplet nuclei; causes infection in 25% of people exposed (conversion of TB skin tests from negative to positive); may remain latent and noninfectious for a lifetime; 10% of those infected may develop tuberculosis disease at some time in their life and be infectious until treatment is initiated
   b. Susceptible populations: aged, the immunosuppressed, immigrant and refugee populations, homeless, those living in poverty in crowded living conditions, infants and children
   c. Symptoms: moderate cough, low-grade temperature, night sweats, weight loss, bloody sputum
   d. Diagnosis: through multilayered system of history of exposure, skin test (PPD—purified protein derivative), chest x-rays, and sputum samples (Table 16-2); preferred screening skin test is the Mantoux Skin Test—0.1 mL of

TABLE 16-2.
Classification System for Tuberculosis

CLASSIFICATION	HISTORY OF EXPOSURE	SKIN TEST	SPUTUM AND X-RAY
0	−	−	−
I	+	−	−
II	+	+	−
III	+	+	+

(Classification II is TB infection, classification III is TB disease. Not shown are classifications IV and V, which refer to stages of TB being treated or post-treatment).

PPD is administered intradermally on the medial aspect of the forearm to achieve a wheal (looks like a mosquito bite); skin test is read 48 to 72 hours later; induration (raised hardened tissue) at the test site is measured, not the redness; results are considered positive:

- ▶ 5 mm or greater: positive skin test in household members or close contact persons; persons with HIV infection
- ▶ 10 mm or greater: positive skin test in foreign-born persons from countries with a high incidence of tuberculosis, high-risk minorities, homeless, medically compromised individuals and those with metabolic disorders
- ▶ 15 mm or greater: positive skin test in all other persons

    e. Treatment: (Table 16-3) isoniazid (INH) is the prophylactic treatment for TB classification II if the client is under 35 years old; bacteriostatic and bactericidal drugs are used in combination when treating TB classification III; TB significantly complicates the crisis of AIDS; treatment of TB in otherwise healthy individuals is complicated with drug-resistant strains

3. Levels of prevention

    a. Primary: teach primary prevention methods; avoid exposure to TB classification III (who are not being treated, who are noncompliant, or who are within the first few weeks of treatment) clients, live a healthy lifestyle, which includes proper diet, rest, and exercise; keep home well ventilated, provide enough space per household member; prevent the TB infection (classification II) from becoming the TB disease (classification III), follow a regimen of prophylaxis with INH

    b. Secondary: increase the number of sites offering TB screening, diagnosis, treatment, medications, counseling and referral services; improve access to comprehensive ser-

TABLE 16-3.
Common Tuberculosis Drugs

FIRST-LINE DRUGS	SECOND-LINE DRUGS	ALTERNATIVE DRUGS
Isoniazid (INH)	Cycloserine	Kanamycin
Rifampin (rifampicin)	Ethionamide	Amikacin
Rifamate (rifampin and INH)	Para-amino salicylate (PAS)	Capreomycin
Pyrazinamide		Ciprofloxacin HCl
Ethambutol		Ofloxacin
Streptomycin		Clofazimine

vices; case management by providers needs to conform to CDC recommendations of medical treatment, follow-up strategies that ensure cure, such as Directly Observed Therapy (DOT), which ensures compliance with drug treatment regimen; notification, TB skin testing, diagnosis, and treatment of family members and other close contacts as needed

c. Tertiary: expand contact tracing efforts; promote rehabilitative and reconstructive care for a high quality of life; continue primary prevention methods

F. Vaccine-Preventable Diseases

1. History

a. In the United States, immunizations have been available since the 1800s to control communicable diseases.

b. Smallpox was the first communicable disease controlled by a vaccine. (World Health Organization eradicated smallpox in the 1980s. We no longer vaccinate against this disease.)

c. In the 1900s, many vaccines became available:

- ▶ DPT (before to World War II)
- ▶ Polio (1950s)
- ▶ Measles, mumps, rubella (1960s)
- ▶ Influenza and pneumonia (1970s)
- ▶ HB and Hib (1980s)
- ▶ Varicella (1990s)

d. United States has been a world leader in requiring childhood immunizations; high levels of immunized children in United States; some people are uneducated as to the value of immunizing their children; constant vigilance by primary and community health providers is necessary

e. **Major outbreaks of communicable disease may occur when the immunization rate drops below 85% (see current immunization schedule in Display 14-1).**

f. Adults should not overlook the need for adult immunizations, such as Td, influenza, pneumonia. Adults should receive prophylactic immunization before travel to certain countries. Also, additional immunizations are required for reentry into the United States after some foreign travel.

2. Levels of prevention

a. Primary: eliminate exposure to people with diseases not immunized against; educate the public regarding the need for immunizations; plan, publicize, and implement immunization campaigns; accessible immunizations (cost, time of day, location, transportation considerations)

    b.   Secondary: early recognition of symptoms; prompt diagnosis and treatment including isolation to prevent spread to unimmunized; contact investigation and case finding

    c.   Tertiary: long-term follow-up as needed; rehabilitative services (polio) as needed; continue with primary prevention practices

G.   Newly Identified and Reemerging Diseases

    1.   Newly identified and reemerging communicable diseases

        a.   Ebola: a viral disease originating in 1976 in the Sudan and Zaire; characterized by sudden onset of fever, malaise, myalgia, and headache, followed by pharyngitis, vomiting, diarrhea, maculopapular rash, hemorrhages, and central nervous system changes; transmitted by close contact with the infected; in Africa, case fatality rate has ranged from 50% to nearly 90%

        b.   Dengue fever: from group B arbovirus transmitted by the mosquito; an acute febrile disease; characterized by sudden onset, headache, fever, prostration, joint and muscle pain, lymphademopathy, rash

        c.   Cholera: an acute infection characterized by profuse watery diarrhea and vomiting; produces severe loss of fluids and electrolytes, muscle cramps, oliguria, dehydration, and collapse; death can occur rapidly due to dehydration and shock; treat by vigorous replacement of fluid and electrolytes; tetracycline given early is effective in killing the causative organism; prevention—give cholera vaccine; where cholera is endemic, avoid drinking unboiled or untreated water, using ice in beverages, eating raw or partially cooked fish, shellfish, uncooked vegetables or unpeeled fruits; between 1911 and 1973, only two reported cases in the Western Hemisphere; by 1994, 950,000 cases reported in 21 countries in the Western Hemisphere, including the United States, primarily Louisiana and Texas

        d.   *Escherichia coli (E coli)*. The colon bacillus. Some strains cause more damage than others. EHEC strains recognized since 1982 cause outbreaks of hemorrhagic colitis; can cause hemolytic-uremic syndrome; children under 5 years of age are at greatest risk of developing the hemolytic-uremic syndrome; prevention includes: managing slaughterhouse operations to minimize contamination of meat by animal intestinal contents; irradiation of beef, especially ground beef; cook beef adequately; protect public water supplies; ensure adequate hygiene in child care centers; frequent handwashing with soap and water is most important

2. Levels of prevention
    a. Primary: eliminate exposure to people with the diseases; educate those traveling in areas where the diseases are endemic regarding the need for precautions; eliminate mosquito breeding reservoirs
    b. Secondary: early recognition of symptoms; prompt diagnosis and treatment including isolation to prevent spread to others; contact investigation and case finding
    c. Tertiary: long-term follow-up as needed; rehabilitative services as needed

III. Levels of Responsibility in Communicable Disease Control

A. International: Work of World Health Organization, UNICEF, CARE, Peace Corps, and other international health organizations needs support in the form of political cooperation and financial resources; mission includes education, surveillance, diagnosis and treatment, and evaluation of efforts to prevent, control, and eliminate communicable diseases

B. Federal: National Institutes of Health, CDC, and the US Public Health Service promote the health of the nation through research, surveillance, diagnostic and treatment services, health services to specific populations; education and training of professionals; grants to states and to groups and individuals involved in health-related research; they act as a resource to states

C. State: State departments of health provide resources to the state in the form of laboratory services, research grants, educational material, and training programs; states gather statistics on diseases occurring in the state and maintain surveillance programs

D. Local: Local or regional health departments work in cooperation with the state and federal levels to protect populations; services are more direct, in that they provide comprehensive communicable disease clinics (TB, STD, immunizations); educate local professionals and the public; deliver specific services funded by the state, such as flu clinics

E. Personal: Individuals have a responsibility to be informed citizens and to focus their self-care activities at the primary level of prevention, which includes maintaining immunization levels and knowing when to seek medical care for unusual or unfamiliar signs and symptoms.

Bibliography

Benenson, A. S. (Ed.).(1995). *Control of communicable diseases manual* (16th ed.). Washington, DC: American Public Health Association.

Centers for Disease Control. (1993). Special Focus: Surveillance for STDs. *Morbidity and Mortality Weekly Report, 42* (No. SS-3).

Centers for Disease Control. (1995). Summary—Cases of specified notifiable disease, United States, cumulative, week ending December 24, 1994 (51st week). *Morbidity and Mortality Weekly Report, 43* (Nos. 51 & 52):962

Grimes, D. E., & Grimes, R. M. (1995). Tuberculosis: What nurses need to know to help control the epidemic. *Nursing Outlook, 43*: 164–173.

Spradley, B. W., & Allender, J. A. (1996). *Community health nursing: Concepts and practice.* (4th ed.). Philadelphia: Lippincott-Raven.

Stanhope, M., & Lancaster, J. (1992). *Community health nursing: Process and practice for promoting health* (3rd ed.). St. Louis: Mosby–Year Book.

US Department of Health and Human Services. (1991). *Healthy people 2000: National health promotion and disease prevention objectives.* DHHS Publication No. (PHS) 91-50212. Washington, DC: Author.

STUDY QUESTIONS

1. A nonhuman agent that actively carries disease organisms to humans is a(n):
   a. Incubator
   b. Vector
   c. Vaccine
   d. Immunization

2. Which of the following is a barrier to communicable disease control?
   a. Inadequate supply of vaccines to administer
   b. Provider lack of knowledge regarding communicable diseases
   c. Client noncompliance with treatment schedules
   d. Old and ineffective immunization materials

3. An example of primary prevention in communicable disease control is:
   a. Screen for disease
   b. Isolation and quarantine
   c. Initiate treatment
   d. Administer immunizations

4. According to the CDC, in 1994 the one reportable communicable disease with the largest numbers in the United States was:
   a. Gonorrhea
   b. AIDS
   c. Tuberculosis
   d. Syphilis

5. Food-borne diseases can escalate into situations with severe consequences. Preventing food-borne diseases at the secondary level of prevention includes:
   a. Replacing lost fluids
   b. Washing foods that will be eaten raw
   c. Cooking meat products thoroughly
   d. Providing supportive care

6. An important thing to remember about vector-borne diseases is that:
   a. Vector-borne diseases do not occur in industrialized countries
   b. Rats are a major vector and there are only mice in the United States
   c. Eliminating insect breeding areas helps control vector-borne diseases
   d. Vector-borne diseases are a minor community health problem

7. Since AIDS was first identified in 1981, other sexually transmitted diseases:
   a. Significantly decreased in number
   b. Continue to exist in large numbers
   c. Do not respond to treatment
   d. Are no longer focused on

8. Tuberculosis is a disease that has been around for centuries. Presently, tuberculosis is:
   a. A dwindling community health problem
   b. Resurging as a major community health concern
   c. Occurring mainly in the AIDS population
   d. Rarely treated because it is not communicable

9. A client with tuberculosis, classification II, is considered:
   a. Noninfectious, negative chest x-ray, but has a positive skin test
   b. Infectious, with a positive chest x-ray and sputum
   c. No history of exposure, skin test is negative, no further tests are conducted
   d. History of exposure, negative skin test, with no further tests

10. Outbreaks of *E coli* infection have recently been occurring in the United States. Which of the following is true about this infection?
    a. The disease is mild, more of a nuisance, especially in children under age 5
    b. Irradiating beef causes the infection and should be discontinued
    c. Imported foods are the major cause and need more stringent monitoring
    d. Hemolytic-uremic syndrome can occur and cause death in the young

ANSWER KEY

1. *Correct response: b*
Answer choices **a, c,** and **d** are not correct responses.
Knowledge/NA/NA

2. *Correct response: c*
Answer choices **a, b,** and **d** are incorrect. Vaccine supplies are adequate, providers are knowledgeable about communicable diseases, and immunization materials are kept up to date and effective.
Comprehension/Health Promotion/Assessment

3. *Correct response: d*
Answer choices **a** and **c** are examples of secondary prevention. Answer choice **b** is an example of tertiary prevention.
Analysis/Health Promotion/Implementation

4. *Correct response: a*
There were almost 73,000 cases of AIDS reported, 22,000 cases of tuberculosis, and 22,000 cases of syphilis; however, there were 388,000 cases of gonorrhea, making it the most frequently reported communicable disease.
Comprehension/Physiologic/Analysis

5. *Correct response: a*
Answer choices **b** and **c** are examples of primary prevention.
Answer choice **d** is an example of tertiary prevention.
Analysis/Health Promotion/Implementation

6. *Correct response: c*
Vector-borne diseases occur in all countries; rats are a major vector and occur in the United States; vector-borne diseases are not minor. Many significant illnesses are related to vectors.
Analysis/Health Promotion/Evaluation

7. *Correct response: b*
Sexually transmitted diseases continue to be a major community health problem, the numbers remain high, and they respond well to treatment—making answer choices **a, c,** and **d** incorrect.
Analysis/Health Promotion/Planning

8. *Correct response: b*
TB is not dwindling. It is resurging, especially among immigrant and refugee populations, homeless, aged, infants, and among those with AIDS. TB infection is not communicable; TB disease is. Both levels are treated with the multiple antituberculosis drugs that have existed since the 1940s.
Analysis/Safe Care/Planning

9. *Correct response: a*
Answer choice **b** describes classification III.
Answer choice **c** describes classification 0.
Answer choice **d** describes classification I.
Analysis/Health Promotion/Implementation

10. *Correct response: d*
E coli outbreaks should be considered serious. Young children are especially vulnerable to hemolytic-uremic syndrome, which can occur when infected with *E coli* from foods grown and processed in the United States. Irradiating beef, frequent handwashing, washing fruits and vegetables in clean water, and cooking meats thoroughly assist in eliminating this community health problem.
Application/Health Promotion/Implementation

Home Health
Nursing Review

Home Health Care—Past, Present, and Future

I. Early Beginnings of Home Health Care
A. A Common Beginning

    1. Public health nursing

        a. Public health nursing as a nursing discipline began through the efforts of Lillian Wald in the late 1800s. Wald began the Henry Street Settlement House, a social service agency, which provided social services and health education. These services were conducted by trained nurses.

        b. The Henry Street Settlement House served the poor immigrant population in New York City. In-home public health services were initially an outreach of the services provided by the agency. Some families were so needy the nurses engaged in personal care, cooking, house cleaning, shopping, and watching children

        c. Nurses delivered "hands-on" services in the clients' homes. Although physicians made regular home visits to the more affluent people, the public health nurse reached the needs of many others.

        d. The public health nurses' holistic services were well received. The overwhelming number of needs, however, caused a strain on the nurse's time and model of care. Nurses began to teach the client and family to provide care. Teaching focused on groups of clients, and visits were to the most ill or highest-risk clients.

e. This model of public health nursing was practiced in urban and rural settings through World War II.

f. **After World War II, public health nursing became more focused on primary prevention and aggregate care to the well, differentiating it from home health nursing.**

2. Home health nursing

a. Early services in the United States were organized and administered by lay people in the late 1800s.

b. In 1877, the Women's Branch of the New York City Mission became the first agency to employ a graduate nurse to deliver home care.

c. The Visiting Nurse Service of New York City, established in 1893 by Lillian Wald and Mary Brewster, was the first private home nursing service.

d. In 1898, the Los Angeles Health Department became the first official agency offering visiting nurse care.

e. **In 1900, home care became the dominant form of nursing. Students trained in hospitals but worked in the community. At this time, public health nursing was not differentiated from home care nursing.**

f. In 1909, the Metropolitan Life Insurance Company began a home nursing service for its New York City policyholders. It was the model for other insurance companies by 1920.

g. **Before World War II, physicians were actively involved in home care; however, the war created a physician shortage and clients began coming to physicians. This created a gap in home care that was filled by growing numbers of visiting nurse associations.**

h. In 1947, the first hospital-based home care program began as a service of Montefiore Hospital in New York City. The program used a team approach and created the first paraprofessional to deliver home care services (a person trained to cook, clean, run errands, and do simple personal care services). By 1958, additional services were added to the program, such as x-ray services, nutritional education, and physical therapy.

i. Many of these scattered programs had financial difficulties. They either relied on donations, service fees, or provided free care. Medicare and Medicaid changed the home health scene in 1966.

3. Medicare/Medicaid (1966)

a. **Medicare brought about changes in payment source, client eligibility, and provision and purpose of care.**

b. Before this federal payment system, physicians did not direct home care. On their own, nurses successfully provided home care to the sick, disabled, and children.

c. Medicare was to act as a gatekeeper of services delivered in the home, requiring physicians to direct the care.

d. **Medicare determines the eligibility, frequency, and type of home care service needed for the client. This gives home care a more narrow focus, becoming a medical-based model of practice.**

e. **During the early years, home health care included health promotion, health teaching, and holistic family care. These are now the focus of public health nursing. Home health care radically changed its focus because of the medical-based practice initiated by Medicare.**

B. **Taking Hold as a Separate Discipline**

1. A slow beginning in the 1970s

a. Some proprietary home health agencies (free-standing for-profit agencies) were not able to develop the service, scope, and complexity required by Medicare. The total number of home care agencies declined in the late 1960s.

b. This led to the growth of official agencies (supported by tax dollars and mandated to offer specific services, such as health departments) and hospital-based home health agencies (extensions of the hospital's services). The greatest growth was in hospital-based agencies during the 1970s.

2. Expansion in the 1980s

a. Proprietary agencies increased in the 1980s when it was ensured that Medicare would pay for home care services. The prospective payment system of diagnostic-related groups (DRGs) set limits on hospital stay, increasing the population who needed home care.

b. It was evident by the 1980s that the home care movement would continue to grow, requiring an increase in skilled nurse practitioners, other professionals, and paraprofessionals (Display 17-1).

3. Challenges of the 1990s

a. Financial structural changes; managed care, more strict service guidelines

DISPLAY 17-1.
Number of Home Care Agencies 1989–1995*

YEAR	NUMBER OF HOME CARE AGENCIES
1989	11,097
1990	11,765
1991	12,433
1992	12,497
1993	13,959
1994	15,027
1995	17,561

(National Association for Home Care, 1995)

    b.   Home care has grown five times faster than the average health industry and accounts for more than 6% of health service jobs. (growing 16.4% annually in the years 1988–1993) (Freeman, 1995).

    c.   Certain changes affect the need for home care services, such as an increase in older clients with multiple chronic illnesses, people living with AIDS (PLWA), hospice and other high-risk clients, ill infants and children, psychiatric clients, and the clients leaving the hospital earlier.

    d.   Care providers need intense orientation, "retooling," and high level skill development to move from acute care and public health settings to the home. The prized asset in the 1990s is knowledge, and home health nursing is considered a high-knowledge industry (Dittbrenner, 1996).

II. The Present Home Health Care System

  A. **Financial Factors**

     1. Medicare: most influential factor on home care

        a.   Focuses on sick care based on reimbursement regulations; creates physician-directed care; determines client eligibility; determines visit frequency and types of service; reimburses for skilled care only

        b.   Places emphasis on paperwork and detailed documentation; creates a need to address reimbursement issues and not just professional care guidelines and standards of care (Harris, 1994)

        c.   Offers 40% of all home care services to clients over 65 who receive 78% of the visits; Medicare reimbursement is important to the solvency of most home health agencies

    d.   A federal program that provides the same benefits to all people who are Medicare eligible (over 65 or permanently disabled), regardless of the state of residence

  2. Medicaid

    a.   Provides for home health care services to the medically indigent of all ages; supplements Medicare in the poor, elderly, or permanently disabled; still must meet criteria for home care for the homebound

    b.   **Allows similar services to Medicare; the state manages the program and provides different coverage in each state**

  3. **Managed care**

    a.   Definition: "a comprehensive approach to health care delivery that encompasses planning and coordination of care, patient and provider education, monitoring of care quality and cost control" (AMCRA, 1995)

    b.   The three main types of managed care organizations (Display 17-2)

    c.   Includes private health insurers, health maintenance organizations, as well as Medicare and Medicaid

    d.   **Health care costs are high; managed care is a significant force in health care, may even be the dominant player in the health care market.**

    e.   For home care and hospice providers, managed care means complicated standards, operation procedures, negotiations, and competition.

DISPLAY 17-2.
Types of Managed Care Organizations

Health Maintenance Organizations (HMOs)

Offers enrollees comprehensive health coverage for hospital and physician services for a prepaid, fixed fee; enrollees must choose among providers; a primary physician normally controls and manages health care services delivered.

Point-of-Service Organizations (POSs)

This system has a network of providers who provide services for a discounted cost; enrollees normally have a primary care physician who refers the enrollee to specialists; enrollees who go outside the system pay more for services; offers more flexibility than the HMO model.

Preferred Provider Organizations (PPOs)

Similar to the POS system except there is no primary care physician who needs to be consulted for out-of-network referrals; costs more to go outside the network for services; is the most flexible of the three managed care models.

B.　Population Changes

1.　Acuity

a.　Acuity is higher among the home care population in the 1990s vs the previous years of the home care movement.

b.　Increased numbers of technology-dependent clients in the home; more resource-intensive clients; longer periods of service needed for complex and chronic illnesses

2.　Age

a.　Home care clients are getting older—significant increase in those over age 85, the fastest growing segment of the population

b.　Older clients are more frail and have a multiplicity of diagnoses and needs.

c.　Transportation, companionship, home repairs, and so forth are not presently provided by home care agencies and are not covered by most insurers, yet these are needs older persons have in common.

3.　Diagnoses

a.　Advances in medicine and treatment modalities enhance survival and longevity, creating a population that in the past succumbed to their illnesses, such as clients with AIDS, end-stage renal disease, and many cancers.

b.　Clients experience very short hospital stays or receive their treatment or surgeries in outpatient settings with follow-up by home health personnel. (Some postpartum women stay in the hospital for less than 24 hours. A home health nurse may make a home visit the next day to assess and teach as needed, but this service is not available to all women; early discharge laws are changing due to the high-risk nature of "drive-by" deliveries.)

C.　Professional Organizations

1.　National Association of Home Care (NAHC)

a.　Proactive group whose mission is to improve the quality of home health care

b.　Informs and inspires home care and hospice care providers in the community

c.　Provides a bevy of direct services to members, including publication of *Caring* magazine and monthly newsletters

d.　Influences significant others who may have an impact on the home care industry (legislature, media, insurers)

2.　American Nurses Association Standards of Home Health Nursing Practice (Display 17-3)

3.　Additional organizations

a.　Council of Home Health Agencies and Community Health Service, the National League for Nursing

DISPLAY 17-3.
ANA Standards of Home Health Nursing Practice*

Standard I. Organization of Home Health Services All home health services are planned, organized, and directed by a master's-prepared professional nurse with experience in community health and administration.

Standard II. Theory The nurse applies theoretical concepts as a basis for decisions in practice.

Standard III. Data Collection The nurse continuously collects and records data that are comprehensive, accurate, and systematic.

Standard IV. Diagnosis The nurse uses health assessment data to determine nursing diagnoses.

Standard V. Planning The nurse develops care plans that establish goals. The care plan is based on nursing diagnoses and incorporates therapeutic, preventive, and rehabilitative nursing actions.

Standard VI. Intervention The nurse, guided by the care plan, intervenes to provide comfort; to restore, improve, and promote health; to prevent complications and sequelae of illness; and to effect rehabilitation.

Standard VII. Evaluation The nurse continually evaluates the client's and family's responses to interventions in order to determine progress toward goal attainment and to revise the data base, nursing diagnoses, and plan of care.

Standard VIII. Continuity of Care The nurse is responsible for the client's appropriate and uninterrupted care along the health care continuum, and therefore uses discharge planning, case management, and coordination of community resources.

Standard IX. Interdisciplinary Collaboration The nurse initiates and maintains a liaison relationship with all appropriate health care providers to ensure that all efforts effectively complement one another.

Standard X. Professional Development The nurse assumes responsibility for professional development and contributes to the professional growth of others.

Standard XI. Research The nurse participates in research activities that contribute to the profession's continuing development of knowledge of home health care.

Standard XII. Ethics The nurse uses the code for nurses established by the American Nurses Association as a guide for ethical decision making in practice.

*(ANA, 1986)

    b. National Home Care Council
    c. National Association of Home Health Agencies
    d. Assembly of Outpatient and Home Care Institutions
    e. American Hospital Association
    f. Specific organizations of professional nursing (hospice nurses, community health nurses, and so forth) and other professional disciplines (social work, occupational therapy, speech therapy, and so forth)
    g. American Nurses' Credentialing Center (ANCC) credentials nurses in over 25 specialty areas including home health nursing

III. The Future in Home Health Care and Nursing
A. Growth
    1. Demographic trends

      a. **Home care will have to grow exponentially to meet the needs of older Americans. Currently, 3.5 million**

US residents are 85 or older. This number will grow to 24 million by the year 2040 (Campion, 1994).

b. Home care industry has grown steadily since the 1980s with all indications that it will continue to do so in response to changes in financing health care and the aging population.

2. Projected needs

a. **Recruitment, training, retention and skill updating of professional and paraprofessional personnel**

b. **Gap-filling community-based services**

c. **Coordination of home care, housing, and health services**

d. **Incentives for consumer and community participation in planning, organizing, and operating home-delivered services**

e. **Integration of formal and informal services**

f. **New funding sources to cover increasing costs**

g. **Simplification of budgetary allocation and service reimbursement procedures**

3. Technological changes

a. Computerized record-keeping systems: eliminates "hard" copies of client charts; changes nurses and others record-keeping style and time demands

b. Client monitoring and medication delivery systems: dramatic changes in technology that allow for patient-activated medication administration for pain relief; smaller and more efficient blood glucose testing and cardiac monitoring systems

c. Portable diagnostic services: laboratory analysis at home, such as blood analysis once done in laboratories

d. Home telemedicine: care brought to the home through interactive video technology—"video visits." Testing this technology indicates it keeps clients at home, reduces emergency room visits, rehospitalization, and institutionalization.

B. Governance Models

1. Hospital-based home health agencies will continue to expand and be used as a marketing tool to entice the client back to that hospital if hospitalization is needed again.

2. Proprietary home health agencies: will continue to grow; may have services contracted by managed care organizations; changes may be needed in organization, standards and services to meet the outcome expectations of the managed care organization

3. Combination agencies: official agencies combine home health services with their public health services; money generated from home health visits subsidize the "free" or low-cost public health services offered

4. Health maintenance organizations: managed care organizations will offer their own home health services

C. Financial Reimbursement

1. Possible changes revolve around increased quality of care; outcome measurements; cost savings
   a. Quality of care: health outcomes and client satisfaction
   b. Outcome measurements: organizational changes occur as providers change to meet demands and requirements of funding sources
   c. Cost savings: outcomes; clinical pathways; intensive services per visit expected with cost savings as the goal

2. Financial restrictions
   a. Pressure to accomplish clinical goals in fewer visits
   b. Focus on teaching caregiving skills to others; monitoring clients from a central location, relying on caregivers or the client to provide the care or to engage in more complex self-care practices
   c. Renewed interest in including informal and voluntary community agencies in caregiving

D. Effects on the Role of the Home Health Nurse

1. Case management role
   a. Increased demand on the home health nurse as a case manager in a managed care environment with more acutely and chronically ill clients
   b. Additional paraprofessionals on the home health team to meet the activities of daily living such as bathing, dressing, and eating (ADL) and instrumental ADLs such as telephoning, shopping, and cooking (IADL) of an aging home care population
   c. Interprofessional collaboration skills will be required of the home health nurse.

2. Special populations managed at home
   a. Technology-dependent clients of all ages will be cared for at home in larger numbers demanding a nurse with well-developed technological skills.
   b. The aged in society (those over age 85) will increasingly need home care services; knowledge of gerontology will be essential
   c. People living with AIDS (PLWA) will increasingly be receiving life-prolonging services at home.

d.   New and resurging diseases demand knowledge of communicable diseases once thought controlled or not before seen in the United States

e.   Use of universal precautions is no longer the ideal but the minimum level of safety for home health nurses.

Bibliography

AMCRA Foundation (1995). *1994–1995 Managed care overview.* Washington, DC: Author

American Nurses Association (1986). *Standards of home health nursing practice.* Washington, DC: Author.

Campion, E. W. (1994). The oldest old. *New England Journal of Medicine, 333:* 18–19.

Dittbrenner, H. (1996). Employment outlook: Put on your sunglasses. *Caring, 5:* 10–12.

Freeman, L. (1995). Home-sweet-home health care. *Monthly Labor Review, 118*(3): 3–12.

Harris, M. D. (1994). Home healthcare nursing is alive, well, and thriving. *Home Healthcare Nurse, 12*(3): 17–20.

National Association for Home Care (1995). *Basic statistics about home care 1995.* Washington, DC: Author.

Rice, R. (1996). *Home health nursing practice: Concepts & application* (2nd ed.). St. Louis: Mosby.

Spradley, B. W., & Allender, J. A. (1996). *Community health nursing: Concepts and practice.* (4th ed.). Philadelphia: Lippincott-Raven.

Stanhope, M., & Knollmueller, R. N. (1996). *Handbook of community and home health nursing* (2nd ed.). St. Louis: Mosby.

Stanhope, M., & Lancaster, J. (1992). *Community health nursing: Process and practice for promoting health* (3rd ed.). St. Louis: Mosby–Year Book.

STUDY QUESTIONS

1. Home health nursing is a discipline of nursing that is:
   a. Growing slowly and hires very few nurses
   b. Having the same effect on the health care delivery as it always has
   c. Fast growing and hires a significant number of nurses
   d. A declining form of nursing care that still needs to be considered

2. Lillian Wald is remembered for her work in:
   a. Establishing public health and home health nursing
   b. Improving nursing care services in the hospitals of her day
   c. Increasing the educational requirements for graduate nurses
   d. Bringing new graduates into the community to work

3. Physicians delivered care in the home before World War II. During the war, clients began to come to the physician instead. What caused this change?
   a. Gas prices increased, and it was more cost-effective for the physicians.
   b. People were moving to rural areas, and doctors had to travel too far.
   c. Many physicians were in the military. The few remaining needed the clients to come to them.
   d. The home environment was no longer an appropriate place for clients to be seen by physicians.

4. Medicare influenced changes in the home care movement by:
   a. Financially reimbursing for all the needs of people receiving home care
   b. Defining client eligibility with physicians directing home care activities
   c. Broadening the definition of home care through its reimbursement system
   d. Creating a state payment system to provide unique coverage in each state

5. The greatest challenges to the home care movement in the 1990s include:
   a. Managing the decreasing numbers of potential clients
   b. Dealing with younger clients who have acute illnesses
   c. Selecting among the highly skilled and prepared home health employees
   d. Financial structural changes that include more strict service guidelines

6. Medicaid influences the services provided to clients by:
   a. Providing home health care services to the medically indigent
   b. Giving incentives to employers for hiring people living in the culture of poverty
   c. Doubling the services in the home over and above what Medicare provides
   d. Providing a local financial program in addition to state and federal programs

7. Managed care is best defined as a(n):
   a. Pattern of visiting clients to save driving time and fuel usage
   b. Efficient system of care to increase the number of home visits made each day
   c. Approach to planning and coordinating care that monitors quality and cost
   d. Individual nurse's way of using time and resources to provide quality care

8. The home care population is changing; a profile of typical home care clients include:
   a. Younger clients with acute illnesses
   b. Chronically ill infants and children
   c. Technology-dependent youth and adults
   d. Older clients with complex chronic illnesses

9. Different governance models exist in home health; the one that is a for-profit and free-standing agency is a:
   a. Combination agency
   b. Proprietary agency
   c. Hospital-based agency
   d. Official agency

10. The *most* important skill of the home health nurse as a case manager includes:
   a. Interprofessional collaboration
   b. Discharge planning
   c. Technological competence
   d. Communicable disease knowledge

ANSWER KEY

1. *Correct response: c*
The other choices do not accurately reflect home health nursing as it is today.
Comprehension/NA/NA

2. *Correct response: a*
Lillian Wald did not work to alter nursing care delivered in hospitals or the educational requirements of new graduates. Nursing graduates at the turn of the century worked in the community after training in hospitals. That was the norm.
Comprehension/NA/NA

3. *Correct response: c*
The alternative responses are not reasons why the change occurred. There were fewer physicians to serve the civilian population, and the change was necessary.
Comprehension/NA/NA

4. *Correct response: b*
In answer choice **a**, Medicare does not cover all the needs of clients. Guidelines are very specific as to what is covered.
Answer choice **c** suggests Medicare has broadened the definition of home care. It has actually narrowed it to a medical-based model of service.
Answer choice **d** indicates Medicare is a state system. It is a federal system with care reimbursed in the same way in each state.
Comprehension/NA/Analysis

5. *Correct response: d*
The numbers of home care clients are increasing. They are older with multiple chronic illnesses. New employees need extensive orientation and skill enhancement.
Analysis/NA/Planning

6. *Correct response: a*
Medicaid supplements Medicare or is the primary payer for the medically indigent. It is a state-managed program, and, through it, selected services are paid for. There are no incentives in the program for agencies to employ specific people.
Comprehension/NA/Analysis

7. *Correct response: c*
The alternative answer choices are good things to consider and will promote quality and cost savings. However, answer choice **c** best defines the present national trend in financial restructuring of the health care delivery system.

8. *Correct response: d*
The home care population is getting older, and their care needs are more complex and often deal with several chronic illnesses at one time. The other groups mentioned in the alternative choices are in the home care population, but not in the numbers that the elderly with chronic illnesses are.
Analysis/NA/Planning

9. *Correct response: b*
Answer choice **a** is an agency that combines an official and a proprietary agency together. It provides home care for a fee and public health services for no fee.
Answer choice **c** is financially associated with a hospital and is not free-standing. It may or may not be for-profit, depending on the mission of the hospital.
Answer choice **d** provides mandated services and is not for-profit.
Comprehension/NA/NA

10. *Correct response: a*
The alternative choices include skills that enhance the role of a home health nurse. However, the *most* important skill is that of interprofessional collaboration—being able to work with other team members to benefit the client with the most timely, highest quality and cost-effective care.
Comprehension/Safe Care/ Implementation

Dimensions of Home Health Care

18

I. Initiation of Home Health Care

   A. Physician's Direction

      1. All home care services are physician directed.

      2. Physicians can order a broad array of home care providers to deliver care in the home (see Section II).

      3. Home care is initiated when a client is to be discharged from an acute care setting or referred from an outpatient setting, has health care needs that can be met at home, meets home care criteria, and care is ordered by a physician.

239

B.   Discharge Planning

1.   Ideally, home care arrangements are made while a client is still hospitalized to promote continuity of care from hospital to home.

2.   Hospitals, rehabilitation facilities, and skilled nursing facilities have discharge planning staff members (nurses or social workers) to coordinate a smooth transition to the next level of care.

3.   A home health agency designates a nurse to coordinate client transition into home care as well; clients are referred by a physician or hospital discharge planner; the home care representative completes an assessment and begins admission into the home care agency if the client desires; it is illegal for a hospital to have an exclusive contract with only one home health agency.

4.   Home health nursing coordinators perform services vital to the marketing and survival of the agency.

II.   Home Health Care Services

A.   Financial Considerations

1.   Third-party payers (insurers) pay for the bulk of home care services (Medicare, Medicaid, and private insurers)

2.   Home health care (personnel, equipment, and supplies), although less expensive than hospital care, can become expensive. Most people cannot afford services for long if it is not covered by insurers.

B.   Personnel

1.   Personnel in home health care are professionals and paraprofessionals; support staff includes secretarial and bookkeeping staff.

2.   Professional staff are state licensed, some with advanced academic degrees and certifications.

3.   Paraprofessionals have training that is basic to their job requirements, laws of the state, and agency needs and expectations.

C.   Durable Equipment

1.   Many home care clients are dependent on an assortment of durable equipment (equipment that is used for a long period of time and can be used again by others, such as wheelchairs, walkers, hospital beds, ventilators, IV poles, and so forth).

2.   Insurers pay for physician-ordered equipment with percentage limitations or a copayment requirement; this allows a client to receive the equipment without paying the full amount; indigent clients may have the total cost covered by being eligible for Medicaid in addition to other insurers.

D.   Supplies

1.   Client supply needs are broad and may include gloves, dressings, irrigation equipment, and disposable incontinence supplies.

2. Supplies used for care that is related to skilled needs are covered in full by insurers or with a small copayment; most insurers do not cover disposable paper products for incontinent clients. Medicaid does; Medicare does not.
3. Medicare covers 100% of dressings used by licensed staff if the home health agency takes them to the home; supplies for skilled needs, taken to homes by durable medical equipment companies (DME), will have a 20% copayment.
4. If supplies are not covered in full, even the small copayment adds up because, large amounts of supplies are often needed and over a long period of time (Display 18-1).

III. Home Health Care Providers
A. Nursing Care Services
    1. Registered Nurses
        a. General practitioner nurses should be well prepared in medical-surgical nursing, gerontology, public health principles, and case management. A bachelor's degree in

DISPLAY 18-1.
Cost of Home Care Supplies to One Family

Marion Smally is 55 and has had multiple sclerosis for 30 years. She has an at-home bookkeeping business and has been ambulatory most of the years since diagnosis but more recently has become homebound, in bed or a wheelchair. Her skin is very sensitive to any trauma occurring when transferring or during periods of incontinence. She frequently has home health care nurses to treat decubitus ulcers occurring on her coccyx or upper thighs and to teach her husband how to change the dressings. Her husband picks up the supplies needed and has kept a record of yearly costs.

ITEM	ANNUAL COST
Disposable pads—12 cartons of 48	12 × 37.64 = 451.68
Disposable incontinence underwear—12 boxes of 72	12 × 58.12 = 697.44
Sterile 4 × 4s—260 boxes of 48	260 × 4.96 = 1289.60
Wound packing gauze—200 bottles of 30 yards	200 × 6.83 = 1366.00
Paper tape—12 boxes of 10 rolls	12 × 28.85 = 346.20
48 bottles of sterile saline	48 × 2.19 = 105.12
24 boxes of latex gloves	24 × 10.25 = 246.00
	Total = $4502.04

Mrs. Smally's health insurance covers 100% of the first $1000 of supplies and 80% of the second $1000 and 50% of anything over $2000. Out-of-pocket expenses for Mrs. Smally are $1451.02 a year. An average of $120 a month has to come out of the family budget just to treat the wounds and occasional incontinence experienced by Marion. Her chronic illness had many additional costs over the last 30 years, including medications, physical therapy, disease-related vision changes and eyeglass needs, wheelchair, furniture and computer adaptations to allow her to continue to work. The dressing and incontinence supplies are a minor portion of the out-of-pocket expenses incurred by this family. The supply costs have been fairly constant for the last 5 years, and Marion is not eligible for Medicare for 7 years.

nursing should be the minimum preparation for home health nursing. However, in many communities, the pool of nurses does not have many bachelor's-prepared nurses. Inservice programs geared to the needs of diploma and associate degree nurses help to prepare them for the demands of the role in home health nursing. Previous work experience in a medical-surgical area as a registered nurse may be required by the home health agency.

b. Advanced practice nurses (clinical nurse specialists or nurse practitioners) are essential to home health agencies delivering specialized services such as enterostomy, wound, or diabetic care; pediatric, geriatric, or psychiatric advanced practice nurses often complement the nursing services needed by the home care population.

c. Special certifications—intravenous, chemotherapy, phlebotomy, phototherapy, and so forth—are offered by the home care agency to standardize skill level of licensed staff and provide safe and high-quality care to clients.

2. Licensed Practical (Vocational) Nurses

a. **Work under the direct supervision of a registered nurse**

b. Deliver independent care to a home care client who has been assessed and opened to the agency for service by a registered nurse; the registered nurse determines that the caregiving needs of the client are within the skill level and scope of practice of an LPN (LVN)

3. Home Health Aides

a. A paraprofessional caregiver who has completed a nursing assistant level course of study that is usually 6 to 12 weeks in length and is supplemented with additional course work in home health care; each state and agency has specific requirements that need to be met by these paraprofessional caregivers

b. Home health aides are supervised by registered nurses, LPNs, or LVNs and provide intermittent personal care services to clients who are receiving professional nursing care and other supplemental therapies

B. Supplemental Therapies

1. Physical Therapy (PT)

a. A physical therapist is either on staff (larger agencies) or contracted for services from hospitals, private PT groups, or individual PTs

b. PT services are ordered by the physician; a home visit is made by the physical therapist for assessment of the client and the home environment

     c.   Services include recommendations for and procurement of home modifications for safety (shower bars, bathtub rails, elevated toilet seat); developing a plan of treatment focused on physical rehabilitation or maximizing strength potential for safety and quality of life related to debilitating diseases or surgical procedures; assessment of clients with supportive equipment such as braces; assessment of clients using walkers and canes for proper technique

     d.   Clients include those with post hip fracture or replacement, other skeletal surgeries or injuries; the frail elderly who need strength training for safety and increased mobility; clients moving toward the use of ambulation aids

     e.   Repeated home visits are limited; it is expected that the home care nurse will reinforce client compliance with the client and caregiver as designated in the treatment plan

     f.   Coordination of care with other professional, paraprofessional, client, and family team members is essential

     g.   Paraprofessionals may be taught exercises by the PT, OT, ST to do with the client.

2. Speech Therapy (ST)

     a.   A speech therapist is either on staff (larger agencies) or contracted for services.

     b.   ST services are ordered by the physician; a home visit is made by the speech therapist for client assessment.

     c.   Services include developing a plan of treatment focused on improvement in oral communication; typical clients are post CVA or have other neurologic processes or injury; exercises are taught to and practiced by the client; activities are reinforced by home care nurses and caregivers; visits occur more frequently by STs than PTs to assess progress and suggest alternative exercises; however, more clients require PT than ST

     d.   Coordination of care with other professional, paraprofessional, client, and family team members is essential.

3. Occupational Therapy (OT)

     a.   An occupational therapist is either on staff (larger agencies) or contracted for services.

     b.   OT services are ordered by the physician; a home visit is made by the occupational therapist for client assessment.

     c.   Services include modifications in the home environment; identification or creation of equipment and adaptive devices that promote client independence that are geared toward the client's new abilities and vocation;

changes are made to accommodate the vocation; assessment of interests in or developing a new vocation within the client's limitations is conducted

d. Coordination of care with other professional, paraprofessional, client, and family team members is essential.

4. Recreational Therapy (RT)

   a. A recreational therapist is usually contracted for services because agencies cannot support a full- or part-time position; limited insurers cover recreational therapy services; a specialty of RT is the play therapist; agencies with a large pediatric population may contract for a play therapist

   b. RT services are ordered by the physician; a home visit is made by the recreational therapist for client assessment.

   c. RTs identify and design recreational activities appropriate for the client's age, interests, and limitations; coordination of efforts are essential with PT, OT, and caregivers; the home care nurses also work with the RT plan

C. **Social Work Services**

1. Social service collaboration is needed to identify the social and emotional problems that negatively impact the client's medical condition, treatment plan, or rate of recovery.

2. Clinical indicators of social service need include:

   a. Ineffective client-caregiver-family-home care team functioning pattern (noncompliance, caregiver stress)

    b. **Suspected child/adult abuse or neglect (nurses are legally mandated reporters of suspected abuse or neglect in most states; a report to child welfare services or the local agency on aging generates the involvement of a social service worker)**

   c. Inadequate income or housing conditions (demonstrated by a lack of resources for basic necessities: food, food storage and cooking facilities, heating, cooling, clothing, telephone, medicines, transportation)

   d. High-tech home care needs

   e. Severe impairments: physical, visual, hearing, mental, emotional

   f. Debilitating or terminal illnesses

   g. Recent amputations, new diagnoses, counseling or community resource needs

   h. Need for long-term care placement

3. Role of social worker in home care

   a. Attends case conferences to coordinate needed social services with other home care services

   b. Acts as a resource to other home care team members

  c. Assists clients and caregivers in resource management to promote continuity of care

  d. Assists with transition from different levels of care to home and long-term care placements as needed

  e. Skilled social worker visits are reimbursed by Medicare if the visits meet Medicare guidelines and are documented appropriately.

IV. The Uniqueness of the Home Setting

 A. Differences From Acute Care Nursing (see Chap 10)

  1. Autonomous practice: works alone in the home; may not see other staff for most of the work day; professional consultation occurs by phone; relies on own skills of assessment, planning, implementation, and evaluation

  2. Uniqueness of the setting: the nurse is a guest in the client's home environment; the nurse is not on his or her "turf"; homes are not all alike; housekeeping or home management styles may distract the nurse, which can affect the quality of care delivered; resources common in the acute care setting are not present

  3. Improvisation: equipment and supplies may be different, in short supply, or absent; the nurse improvises caregiving within the limits of safety using available materials

  4. Clinical assessment: the home care nurse must have well-developed physical assessment skills; high-tech assessment tools in the home are limited; consultation occurs by telephone based on the nurse's findings (technology brings assessment data directly to the physician for immediate decision making—not all home health agencies have access to this technology)

  5. Decision-making skills: essential due to the solo practice; access to others for consultation is limited; decisions are made based on the nurse's assessment

  6. Knowledge of community resources and financial mechanisms is necessary.

  7. Interprofessional collaboration skills are essential to work with multiple agencies in the community.

 B. Differences From Community Health Nursing

  1. Includes physical and high-tech nursing care—wound care; IM and IV medications; treatments; teaching focused on the needs of acutely or chronically ill clients

  2. The home care population is not a well population. The focus is on secondary and tertiary prevention; primary prevention is the focus in community health (see Chap 1)

  3. Most visits are made to the elderly; community health nurses focus primary prevention on high-risk groups, pregnant women, infants, and children

V.   The Nurse's Role
A.   Clinician
1.   Assessment: physical, emotional, environmental, community
2.   Implements a variety of clinical treatments
3.   Client population across the lifespan: with a focus on the aged; gerontologic nursing and chronic illness knowledge essential
4.   Environment changes with each client; able to conduct assessments, provide care, and teach in unique settings

B.   Teacher
1.   Client: teaches self-care management techniques to clients who are acutely and chronically ill; clients have different levels of cognitive abilities, formal educational levels, interest in their health status; teaching techniques need to be adapted to the client's ability and the environment; many clients live alone with no family members or caregivers
2.   Caregivers: if present, are included in the teaching; caregivers frequently need to learn skilled caregiving techniques, such as monitoring IVs, administering IM medication, dressing wounds, and so forth; the nurse must be a talented educator to teach lay people these skills
3.   Ancillary personnel: home health nurses teach home health aides or homemakers to individualize care based on the plan of care for each client
4.   Peers: conducting formal staff inservices and informal information sharing are common expectations of nurses in home care

C.   Collaborator: home care nurses collaborate with professionals and paraprofessionals to provide comprehensive care in the home
1.   Physician: directs home care services
2.   Other home care team members (discussed earlier in Sect. III)
3.   Client pharmacist: assists in coordinating medication regimen; supply age- and ability-appropriate medication containers; deliver medications to the homebound; a resource to the nurse and family for drug interaction information
4.   Community agencies: provide services the client may need (educational material, support groups); as an educational resource to the nurse

D.   Leader: including management and supervision of others
1.   Personal time schedule: home health nurses plan their day separate from shift work and the routine of the acute care setting; efficient use of time is essential to allow adequate visit time and to be a cost-effective employee for the agency; effi-

ciently and safely travels to client's homes; conserves supplies; manages the care of a client caseload

    2. Ancillary personnel: supervises home health aides (Medicare requires that home health aides be supervised; every 2 weeks, a registered nurse makes a supervisory home visit to observe the home health aide providing care and assesses the clients' perception of care)

    3. Students: undergraduate or graduate nursing students use the agency for clinical practice; staff nurses assume a leadership position acting as role models or preceptors for the student's educational experience

    4. New staff members: mentor new staff during orientation and with beginning home health nurses

    5. Documenting care: leadership is demonstrated through concise and thorough documentation that accurately reflects client condition and care provided; agency survival depends on the nurse meeting the documentation expectations reimbursement by fiscal intermediaries

VI. Legal and Ethical Issues in Home Care

A. Employment Considerations (questions for nurses to ask)

    1. Is the nurse an employee of the agency or an independent contractor?

    2. Are the nurses familiar with the type of care and treatment clients require and the equipment that will be used? Are in-service education opportunities provided by the agency?

    3. Does the agency provide proper orientation to the expected role and the responsibilities to the client and the home health agency?

    4. Does the agency provide a safe work environment?

    5. Are the nurses familiarized with state reporting and documentation requirements?

B. Documentation

    1. The cornerstone of the defense of any malpractice claim is complete, accurate, and truthful documentation, which includes:

        a. Objective record keeping

        b. Each entry dated with time of the visit

        c. Entries signed with initial, last name and title

        d. Client name on each page of the chart

        e. Documentation of all client/caregiver teaching

        f. Documentation of noncompliance with treatment plans

        g. Use agency-approved abbreviations

        h. Properly corrected errors in documentation

        i. **Do not rewrite notes, even to obtain reimbursement for the client or agency (this is an unethical practice)**

2. Common areas of liability include client falls, medication errors, faulty equipment, communication and safety problems, inadequate medical response, admitting inappropriate clients into home care

3. All care delivered in the home is physician directed. However, there are exceptions to this general rule:
   a. The order is illegible.
   b. The order is illegal.
   c. Following the order could cause harm to the client.
   d. The order is against the policy of the agency.
   e. The home health nurse is not trained properly or licensed to carry out the order.

4. Valid informed consent of the client and/or the legally authorized substitute decision maker must be obtained before initiating any medical intervention; a copy of this document should be in the client record

C. Incidence Reports

1. Documenting "incidents" (as observed, found, or as a participant) is required by home health agencies; complete and forward incident report to designated agency staff member within 24 hours of the incident

2. These documents are used for risk management and kept within the agency; they may become a part of a legal action only if requested by the plaintiff's attorney

3. Information is factual; avoid statements that affix blame, express opinions, or draw conclusions

4. Document the incident in the client record; do not document that an incident report was completed; the report is kept confidential and in the home health agency; the fact that an incident report has been made is not mentioned in the client record (may call attention to the incident and signal the plaintiff's attorney that a standard of care was not followed) (Display 18-2)

DISPLAY 18-2.
Essential Contents of Incidence Reports

Date, time, and location of incident
Family member notified (name, time, by phone or in person)
Name of physician notified and time
Facts of the occurrence
Direct quotes from the client or other third parties
Assessment of the client, using objective documentation
Action taken

D. **Client Rights and Responsibilities**
  1. When opening a new case to the home health agency, the nurse reviews the agency "patient rights and patient responsibilities" form with the client; it follows a standard pattern of patient rights and responsibilities similar to those used in acute care agencies
  2. The rights and responsibilities form gives the home health agency a better position to close the case of an abusive or noncompliant client; it informs the client of the courtesy and quality of care they can expect

E. **Patient's Self-Determination Act**
  1. Part of the Omnibus Budget Reconciliation Act (OBRA), effective in 1991
  2. This act allows a competent client to advise others of his or her choices of treatment in the event of future incapacity through a valid living will (a form of advance directive); it indicates the client's wishes in regards to CPR, artificial respiration, and artificial means of hydration and nutrition
  3. A copy of the client's advance directives must be in the client record (or the client is educated concerning the applicable state laws and the agency's policies regarding advance directives) in order for the home health agency to continue to receive Medicare and Medicaid funds

VII. **Improvising Care: the community health nurse who works in home health care has many opportunities to be creative**
  A. Materials and Supplies
    1. Home care services are often carried out with materials and supplies much less sophisticated than in the acute care setting. However, they are as effective and less expensive. Examples include:
       a. A dish pan bought in the grocery store for a diabetic to do foot care
       b. Disposal of used syringes and needles in a coffee can, plastic lid taped to it with a slot for insertion
       c. "Clean" small dressing supplies made by cutting needed sizes from larger dressings
       d. Using a recipe for making normal saline or a replacement supplement for infants (such as Pedialyte) using inexpensive household products
  B. **Environmental Modifications: equipment that is expensive or unavailable can be improvised; home health nurses are familiar with these types of differences from the acute care setting and are not uncomfortable with the differences. Examples include:**
    1. Plywood over steps to make a home wheelchair accessible
    2. Draw sheets made from folded top sheets

3. A flannel-backed plastic tablecloth as a protective barrier between bottom sheet and draw sheet

4. A plastic swivel platter that can be used to bring medicines or dressing supplies within reach

VIII. Infection Prevention and Control (for history and epidemiology, see Chaps 2 and 7)

A. **Maintaining Infection Control**

1. Basic principles of good hygiene, clean nursing care, and sterile nursing procedures are followed in the home.

2. **Wash hands before and after contact with the client; this is essential on every home visit and cannot be overemphasized; handwashing supplies should be brought on the visit; not all homes will have access to the facilities or supplies needed (Display 18-3)**

3. Clients are exposed to fewer foreign organisms at home; when infections occur, they are usually from organisms introduced into their system by others (during dressing changes, catheterization; from an ill caregiver); healthy household members are able to tolerate the household organisms; because a client's health is compromised, the immediate environment needs to be safe and as clean as possible

4. A total home assessment and instruction for safety are conducted with the client, family, and/or caregiver at the beginning of home health care service in many agencies.

5. At home, some treatments treated as "sterile" in acute care settings can be "clean" procedures; they are treated as sterile procedures in acute care settings to protect the client from the casual introduction of organisms from other clients, per-

DISPLAY 18-3.
Recommended Personal Protective Equipment

- ▶ Disposable nonsterile/sterile gloves and utility gloves
- ▶ Disinfectants
  Chemical germicides
  EPA-registered products effective against HIV
  5.25% sodium hypochlorite (household bleach)
- ▶ Masks (CPR, air purifying, goggles)
- ▶ Moisture-proof aprons/gowns, shoe covers, caps
- ▶ Leak-proof and puncture-proof specimen containers
- ▶ OSHA-approved sharps container
- ▶ Liquid soap, soap towelettes, dry hand disinfectants
- ▶ Paper towels
- ▶ Bottled sterile water for eye irritation
- ▶ A change of clothing kept in a plastic bag in the car
- ▶ A nursing bag for supplies
- ▶ Newspaper (as a barrier to place items on in the home)

haps causing a nosocomial (hospital-acquired) infection from contact, droplet, air-borne, or vector-borne transmission (see Chaps 7 and 16)

6. **Personal protective equipment should be provided to the employee by the home health agency (see Display 18-3)**

B. **"Standard Precautions"**

1. Two-tier isolation guidelines developed by the CDC in 1995 called *Standard Precautions:* first tier uses major features of universal precautions and principles of body substance isolation (BSI); second tier uses a disease-specific approach according to mode of transmission

2. "Standard precautions" reflect the Occupational Safety and Health Administration's (OSHA) blood-borne pathogen standard and follows the JCAHO standards for home care; promote handwashing and use of gloves, masks, eye protection, or gowns when appropriate for client contact

all clients should be treated as if they have a communicable disease

3. Body substance isolation from breast milk, blood, feces, urine, droplet or air-borne spray from a cough, tissues, vomitus, wound, or other drainage are standard practices of the home health nurse.

4. Clean-up of spills in the home can be safely handled with a 1:10 ratio of bleach and water solution.

Bibliography

Caie-Lawrence, J., Peploski, J., and Russell, J. C. (1995). Training needs of home healthcare nurses. *Home Healthcare Nurse, 13*(2): 53–60.

Rice, R. (1996). *Home health nursing practice: Concepts and application.* St. Louis: Mosby–Year Book.

Spradley, B. W., & Allender, J. A. (1996). *Community health nursing: Concepts and practice.* (4th ed.). Philadelphia: Lippincott-Raven.

Williams, E. (1995). Understanding social work in the home health care setting. *Journal of Home Health Care Practice, 7*(2):12–20.

STUDY QUESTIONS

1. All home health care services are directed by the:
   a. Home-care coordinator
   b. Physician
   c. Case manager
   d. Discharge planner

2. The core group of service providers in the home care setting include:
   a. Home health aides, nurses, and social workers
   b. Nurses, recreational therapists, and nutritionists
   c. Home health aides, occupational therapists, and pharmacists
   d. Speech therapists, social workers, and nutritionists

3. Durable equipment includes such items as:
   a. Dressings
   b. Gloves and gowns
   c. Wheelchairs
   d. Oxygen tubing

4. A social worker as a professional staff member in a home health agency can assist with successful client recovery goals by:
   a. Making a shared visit with the nurse to assist in personal caregiving
   b. Contributing relevant client social information during case conferences
   c. Consulting with the staff of a skilled nursing facility for several weeks after a home care client is admitted
   d. Supervises the care given by staff delivering special therapies in the home

5. Differences in ⸻home health nursing from the acute care setting include the following concepts:
   a. Physical assessment skills are not as important—the clients are not as ill.
   b. Improvising does not occur in the home as frequently as in the hospital.
   c. Decision-making skills are not used as frequently as in the hospital.
   d. Knowledge of community resources and financial mechanisms is necessary.

6. Differences in home health nursing from nursing in public health agencies include:
   a. Public health nurses focus on primary prevention and do not provide physical nursing care.
   b. The home health population is a healthy population and not as ill as in public health nursing.
   c. Home health clients are younger than clients in public health settings.
   d. Pregnant women, infants, and children make up most of the caseload in home health nursing.

7. Both public health nurses and home health nurses have the following roles as part of their practice. The one role that is the most similar is:
   a. Clinician
   b. Collaborator
   c. Teacher
   d. Leader

8. Documentation of home health care nursing visits must meet the same standards expected in other health care settings, in addition to:
   a. Being understandable to the client and family members
   b. Meeting requirements set by fiscal intermediaries
   c. Rewriting the notes to comply with Medicare guidelines
   d. Absence of any abbreviations in the charting

9. A physician writes an order for one of your clients to take a daily dose of medication that is three times higher than the upper daily limits of that medication according to the most recent edition of a nurses' drug manual. Your best action would be to:
   a. Teach the client side effects to look for and tell them to discontinue the medication if any of the side effects occur
   b. Check with other nurses in the agency to see if this is a new practice or a practice of this one physician

   c. Verify the order with the ordering physician; withhold the medication from the client until clarified

   d. Suggest to the client that family members or caregiver check this order with the physician

10. You are making a home visit to Sara Williams, an 82-year-old woman, 5 weeks after hip fracture. You find her on the bathroom floor with the care-taker attempting to assist her to stand with the help of a neighbor. You provide appropriate assistance, assessment, and follow-up to her physician. However, you also write up an incident report. This document objectively states what you observed and actions taken. The document is:

   a. An official part of the client's chart

   b. A legal document to be forwarded to the client's lawyer

   c. Kept in the agency and used for quality and risk management

   d. Used as the charting of the incident and placed in the client's chart

ANSWER KEY

1. *Correct response: b*
All home care services are ordered and directed by the physician; the other practitioners have responsibilities in carrying out parts of the services to the home care client.
Comprehension/NA/NA

2. *Correct response: a*
Nutritionists, recreation therapists, and pharmacists are not usually considered core staff members in home health agencies. Their professional contributions and opinions are sought by home health agencies either as a consultant or on a contractual basis. Nurses, home health aides, and social workers are hired by home health agencies as core staff members.
Analysis/NA/NA

3. *Correct response: c*
Durable equipment includes those items that are not disposable after use and may be used by the client either by buying or renting the equipment. Items called supplies are disposable after one client's use.
Comprehension/NA/NA

4. *Correct response: b*
Social workers do not assist with personal care in the home nor do they supervise other caregivers. Social work services provided by the home health agency do not follow the client to another setting for long periods of time.
Application/Safe Care/Implementation

5. *Correct response: d*
Answer choices **a, b,** and **c** are incorrect. Physical assessment skills, improvising, and decision-making skills are important in both settings but are needed more in the home care setting due to the autonomous nature of the practice.
Application/Safe Care/Implementation

6. *Correct response: a*
Home health nursing populations are older, have acute and chronic illnesses, and have home health nursing visits because they are ill or injured.
Application/Health Promotion/Implementation

7. *Correct response: c*
The role of teacher is the most alike of the roles mentioned. The home health nurse as clinician provides physical nursing care; collaborates primarily with a team of professionals and paraprofessionals; and the leadership role is with professionals and paraprofessionals within the agency. The public health nurse does not provide personal nursing care; collaborates and is a leader with a broader scope of people in the community.
Comprehension/NA/Analysis

8. *Correct response: b*
Documentation is not completed for the client's understanding, standard medical/nursing terminology is used. It is never appropriate to rewrite documentation. This is an unethical practice. Agency-approved abbreviations are appropriate to use.
Application/Safe Care/Implementation

9. *Correct response: c*
Because this order is so dramatically out of the normal range of doses for this medication, as the client's home health nurse you should withhold the ordered dose until clarified by the physician. Checking with others, having family or caregivers follow up, or suggesting the medication be taken and side effects watched for are dangerous practices that threaten the health, and perhaps the life, of the client while placing decisions in the hands of someone else,

even nonprofessionals. You are the primary professional caregiver and need to follow up with the most restrictive approach to promote client safety.

Application/Safe Care/Implementation

10. *Correct response: c*

The incident report is completed and kept within the agency. Completion of this document is not mentioned in the client's chart, not placed in the chart, not forwarded to the client's lawyer, nor substituted for normal charting. It is an internal document for quality and risk management. Data collected from incident reports assist agencies in changing or reinforcing practices and protocols.

Application/Safe Care/Implementation

Organizational Administration of Home Care Services

19

I. Structural Variances

A. Business "Industry" Terms (Yessne, 1994)

1. Home health services (nursing, therapies, homemaking)
2. Hospice care
3. Home medical equipment, including respiratory therapy
4. Home infusion therapy

B. Home Care Models (Hughes, 1992)

1. High-tech home care. Examples: ventilator-dependent clients, Infusion therapies, AIDS therapies
2. Hospice care: all services (equipment and personnel) that meet the needs of caring for the hospice client family
3. Skilled home health care: Medicare-defined nursing services in the home (may be high-tech, teaching, monitoring health status, and so forth)
4. Low-tech custodial care: those services that promote independence in the elderly and disabled to maintain themselves at home (homemaking, chore services, pet care, shopping, and so forth)

257

C. **Financial Structures (see Chap 17)**
1. Proprietary agencies
2. Voluntary agencies
3. Official agencies

D. **Service Parameters (Handy, 1995)**
1. Home care can encompass over 100 separate services delivered as single services, or clustered into groups, by agencies using one of the above-mentioned structural patterns.
2. Corporate status of the parent entity determines organizational form and service parameters. The services provided reflect:
   a. Philosophy
   b. Marketability
3. Because of the type of home care service provided, state licensure or Medicare certification may be required and significantly impacts administrative structure.
4. A rapidly changing business and service environment forces organizations to modify their internal structures to respond to market forces in order to stay viable. Changes include:
   a. Specialization: selecting one service not well developed by other agencies; doing it well and staying on the "cutting edge" of technology, need, and consumer cost
   b. Segmentation: providing a few selected services
   c. Consolidation: cutting back from a broad array of services and personnel housed in separate buildings and communities; consolidation saves on overhead expenses, such as rent, utilities, secretarial and bookkeeping staff costs
   d. Integration: linking levels of care (vertical integration) or types of services (horizontal integration) in the services provided by the organization

II. **Reimbursement Requirements**
A. **Determinants of Service**
1. Philosophy and mission of organization
   a. Determines the array of services provided
   b. Determines the personnel, numbers, professional category; paraprofessionals; support staff based on the array of services provided
2. Delivery and financing of services
   a. Medicare: all care is physician directed; plan of care developed is detailed and specific to their requirements (presently covers a maximum of 28 hours per week if skilled nursing and home health aide care are combined); uses codes that determine parameters of service; sets limits to services in time and frequency of skilled visits; sets limits to the number and frequency of paraprofessional visits (services are physician recertified every 9 weeks but can be

paid for as long as the services are considered medically reasonable and necessary)

b. Medicaid: coverage differs from state to state; in all states it covers basic home health care, medical equipment, homemaker, personal care, and other services that are not covered by Medicare; eligibility—low income, few savings or other assets; covers what Medicare does not cover for eligible low-income clients; many changes are occurring in Medicare and Medicaid as managed care and health maintenance organizations (HMOs) manage more and more of the health care services

c. Other insurers: have specific requirements for establishing a plan of care; services provided and frequency are different with each insurer and managed care organization

d. Home health organizations offer health care services paid for directly by the client or client's family; services provided are negotiated with the client on a fee-for-service basis; services continue as long as desired by the client or as long as the client is able to pay

B.   Documentation of Services

   1.   Uniqueness of home health documentation

a. Opening a case for service: documentation of services needed is imperative for reimbursement by insurers; responsibility falls to the home health care nurse who opens the case for service; in the acute care setting, decision to admit for service is carried out by an assessment conducted by the physician; in home health, the physician initiates the array of services based on an assessment of need completed by the nurse

b. Documentation occurs at the end of each visit, before the end of the work day

   2.   Indicators of quality documentation

a. Opening a case: client receives information about the home health agency and its services, how to reach the nurse and other agency staff, client rights and responsibilities, advance directives; in some agencies, information about home safety (an assessment of home safety may be conducted with the client or client's caregiver)

b. **Client advocacy: ideal home health care is holistic, the nurse acts as a client advocate (this is documented in the client record); provides services needed by the client and family; initiates referrals for a broad array of services that assist clients in safely remaining at home and with an improved quality of life (eg, meal delivery services, friendly visitor services, chore services, dog grooming, yard maintenance services)**

c. **Client record is an official document: in home health, the documentation forms look different from forms used in acute care settings; using agency format, signatures in appropriate locations, completing all forms, are important principles in quality documentation of home health services (as they are in the acute care setting)**

III. Agency Leadership

   A. Organizational Patterns of Service

   1. Geographic
      a. The community served by the home health agency is divided into sections that assist in organizing a method of service delivery
      b. Geographic decisions may be based on many factors including numbers of clients being served in different sections of the service area, travel distances, nurse's home residence in relation to clients needing service
      c. Geographic distribution of clients provides an organizational system that makes the case assignment process manageable; saves the agency mileage costs (in distance traveled and staff familiarity with one part of the service area); saves nursing time; more visits made each day
      d. Works best in rural agencies where clients and staff may live 20 to 100 miles away from the agency office; weekend and holiday coverage works by having staff assume caregiving in two or three geographic areas and cover for each other on staff days off; clients adjust to only one or two staff member changes, which promotes continuity and quality care

   2. Client Diagnosis
      a. Determines what nurse or home health aide is assigned to the case
      b. Clients have different needs: skill needs differ; time needed to perform skills are different; nurses' skills, abilities, and interests vary; using information about personnel strengths and client need determines case assignment
      c. This system works best in a large agency (with many nurses who have a wide range of experience) serving a geographically small area
      d. Drawbacks: organizing case assignments can be time consuming; weekend coverage needs cannot follow this pattern in most agencies when there is limited staff

   3. Caregiver Specialty
      a. Similar to the client diagnosis system, however an agency may hire nurses with specific skills, just to perform those skills

b. This is the system used in specialty organizations, such as hospices or home infusion agencies

c. Drawbacks: providing specific skilled services increases driving time; mileage costs; limits staff available for hire or increases agency staff training costs

B. Promotion of Quality Care

1. Agency orientation

 a. **Orientation of new staff is critical to providing quality care.**

b. Orientation includes: assessment of nursing skills, review of agency policy and procedure manuals, legal and ethical issues in home care, agency guidelines regarding documentation, universal precautions and safety; assignment of a mentor (clinical preceptor) for guided home visit experiences, development of a case load, and as a continuing professional resource

2. Development of nursing staff

a. Inservice programs: a well-established system of education should be provided by the home health agency; agency has a nurse designated to interview, hire, orient, and inservice the new employee and inservice all staff on a regular basis; in small agencies, this may be a part-time role; in larger agencies, this is the role of the inservice educator

b. Transitioning to home care: orientation for nurses entering home care is focused on promoting independence in the new role; it is individualized to the new employee's needs; a mentor or clinical preceptor (an experienced staff nurse) is assigned to guide the field orientation process and act as a resource to the new employee; a model orientation plan assists in reducing the rate of employee turnover during the first year after hiring

c. Employee career ladder: needed to maintain quality caregiving in home health agencies, includes: pay steps based on increased agency responsibility and leadership, opportunities to mentor new staff; educational advancement such as professional credentials, workshop attendance, university level coursework leading to an advanced degree or a specialized skill

3. Professional advancement

 a. **American Nurses Credentialing Center (ANCC) certification in Home Health Nursing, Community Health Nursing, Gerontology, or other related fields prepares staff nurses for the uniqueness of the setting**

b. Skill-enhancing courses in IV therapy, chemotherapy, ventilator-dependent clients, aerosol therapies, phototherapy (see Chap 20)

     c.   University educational programs: streamlined LPN (LVN) advancement to registered nurse; bachelor's degree programs for diploma and associate degree nurses; master's degree in nursing programs; nurse-practitioner programs; certificate programs in home health nursing offered by universities to "retool" nurses leaving acute care settings for community settings

  4. Standards of care

     a.   National Association for Home Care (NAHC) promotes the standard of in-home health and supportive services by serving as the community's voice before Congress, regulatory agencies, courts, and the media; conducts research; provides legislative, regulatory, and legal assistance; publishes several periodicals

        National Association for Home Care
        519 C Street, NE
        Washington, DC 20002-5809
        (202) 547-7424 Fax: (202) 547-3540

     b.   Home Healthcare Nurses Association (HHNA); started in 1993 as a new specialty nursing organization; serves as a forum for members to discuss and refine the professional, educational, and conceptual aspects of their practice with a goal to foster excellence in practice

     c.   American Nurses Association (ANA) has a long history of improving the standard of nursing care in all nursing settings; is the official voice of nurses in the United States; provides many services and publications

     d.   Unique standards implemented by individual agencies are defined in their documents: mission statements, philosophy, policy and procedure manuals

  5. The informed client

     a.   Advanced directives (see Chap 18)

     b.   Client bill of rights (see Chap 18)

     c.   The home care nurse educates the client or caregiver in self-care and caregiving practices; promotes client involvement in primary caregiver decision making about the client's health—self-advocacy and assertiveness

  6. Agency evaluation methods

     a.   Outcome evaluation: quantitative and qualitative measurements include staff and client outcomes (the observable effects after a treatment, program, or service is introduced and completed); quantitative outcomes—shows increases or decreases in numbers of measurable criteria established by the agency (eg, increased hours of inservice per employee to 2 hours per month from 1 hour a month; decreased urinary tract infection rate from 7% to 4% in 6 months among clients over age 65); qualitative outcomes can be determined by client satisfaction surveys; insurers are requiring measurable criteria that demonstrate positive outcomes as a result of the interventions (nursing care, homemaking service, physical therapy, and so forth) provided and paid for by the insurer

b.   Formative staff evaluation: continuous evaluations that are designed to assist in employee development

c.   Summative staff evaluation: conducted at the end of a predetermined period such as yearly from the date of hire, or every January; used to determine staff education needs, salary increases, continued employment, or dismissal from employment; services are evaluated for appropriateness, cost-effectiveness

d.   Summative client care outcomes: gathered from documented data; information is gathered and future caregiving changes are made based on how well client outcomes were achieved

IV.   Nursing Leadership in Home Care Agencies
A.   Organizational Structure
1.   Nursing organizational structures in home health agencies do not have many levels of nursing administration (Display 19-1).

a.   Most nurses are in staff positions.

b.   Additional nursing positions may include inservice educator, supervising nurse(s), the nursing director of the agency.

c.   Agencies are usually small in comparison to acute care settings; opportunities for promotion to a management position for the staff nurse are not as great.

DISPLAY 19-1.
Home Health Nursing Organizational Structure

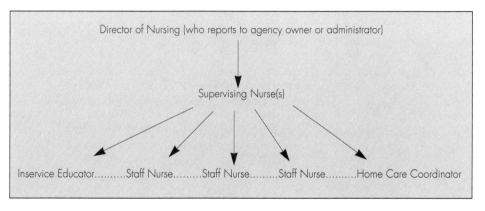

Director of Nursing (who reports to agency owner or administrator)

Supervising Nurse(s)

Inservice Educator..........Staff Nurse.........Staff Nurse.........Staff Nurse..........Home Care Coordinator

        d.   Agencies are growing as more acute care is being delivered in homes; organizational structures may become more complex.

    2.   Nursing care is a major part of the services home health agencies provide; quality of nursing services promote agency recognition, acceptance and leadership in the community and is reflective in the success of the agency.

B.   **Quality Management**

    1.   Total Quality Management (TQM)

        a.   Management approach to long-term success through customer satisfaction

        b.   Continuous system of support and analysis to provide the highest quality of care possible

        c.   System includes work environment, staff qualifications, markers that determine client outcomes, client satisfaction.

        d.   Nursing is a part of the total quality management (TQM) program of an agency.

    2.   The Nurse's Role

        a.   Availability and quality of nursing staff orientation, inservice opportunities, safe and healthy work environment, educational opportunities, availability of appropriate supplies and services to supplement nursing care

        b.   Well-documented care enhances data collection to determine if standards of care have been met.

        c.   Planning and implementation of a system of nursing care review that fits in with the TQM program of the agency

        d.   **Development of an environment that fosters an attitude among nursing staff that each nurse is responsible for providing the highest quality of care possible to assigned clients**

BIBLIOGRAPHY

Handy, J. (1995). Alternative organizational models in home care. *Journal of Gerontological Social Work, 24*(3/4), 49–65.

Hughes, S. (1992). Home care: Where we are and where we need to go. In Ory, M., & Duncker, A. (Eds.). *Home care for older people.* Newbury Park, CA: Sage Publications.

Spradley, B. W., & Allender, J. A. (1996). *Community health nursing: Concepts and practice.* (4th ed.). Philadelphia: Lippincott-Raven.

Yessne, P. (1994). Home health today (part I). *Home Health Business Report, 1,* 13–14.

ANSWER KEY

1. *Correct response: a*

The other terms apply to a population served, one particular service, and the additional supplies agencies have on hand for the nurses when home visits are made to homes without sufficient supplies.

Comprehension/Safe Care/Assessment

2. *Correct response: c*

The four models of care provide different levels of care based on client need: high-tech, low-tech, skilled home health, and hospice care. Within these models, different aged populations are served with different types of service needs. Medicare and Medicaid may pay for services provided within the different models.

Comprehension/Safe Care/Assessment

3. *Correct response: d*

Answer choices **a, b,** and **c** describe consolidation, integration, and segmentation, respectively, the three other modifications to agency internal structure.

Comprehension/Safe Care/Assessment

4. *Correct response: b*

Answer choice **a** better describes the Medicaid program.

In answer choice **c,** all home care services are directed by a physician, making physician care essential to home care services.

In answer choice **d,** home health aide services are financially covered under Medicare but in conjunction with skilled nursing services. Medicare does not cover home health aide services if this is the only service the client needs.

Comprehension/Safe Care/Assessment

5. *Correct response: b*

Charting must be completed daily but the need to chart during care is not as great as in the acute care setting. The other answer choices are the same for acute care settings as well as in home care.

Application/Safe Care/Implementation

6. *Correct response: a*

Answer choices **b** and **c** are not as cost-effective for such a rural agency as described.

Answer choice **d** is not one of the considerations in organizational patterns of service.

Application/Safe Care/Implementation

7. *Correct response: c*

Answer choices **a** and **b** are the same and work better in suburban or rural settings.

Answer choice **d** is not one of the considerations in organizational patterns of service.

Application/Safe Care/Implementation

8. *Correct response: d*

Answer choices **a, b,** and **c** are examples of important orientation needs and outcomes to decrease staff turnover.

Application/Safe Care/Implementation

9. *Correct response: b*

The NAHC does not accredit home health agencies nor train new nurses.

Answer choice **d** better describes the mission of the Home Healthcare Nurses Association (HHNA).

Comprehension/Safe Care/Assessment

10. *Correct response: c*

Client outcomes are the measurable criteria of caregiving, and good outcomes are the goal of any quality management program. The other answer choices are important but are not the goal of a quality management program.

Analysis/Safe Care/Evaluation

Home Health Care

20

I. **Maternal and Infant Care**
   A. High-Risk Pregnancy
   B. Postpartal Complications
   C. Maternal/Newborn Follow-up
   D. Infant Illness
II. **Child Care**
   A. Acute Illness
   B. Chronic Illness
III. **Adult and Older Adult Care**
   A. Acute Illness
   B. Chronic Illness
   C. Alterations From Basic Needs
   D. Nursing Diagnoses
IV. **Supplies and Equipment**
   A. Intravenous Equipment
   B. Dressing Distributors
   C. Dressing Supplies
   D. Oxygen Therapy
V. **Technology in the Home**
   A. Pumps
   B. Ventilators
   C. Phlebotomy
   D. Phototherapy
   E. Nutritional Supplementation
   F. Elimination Technology
   G. New or Experimental Therapies
VI. **The Nursing Process**
   A. Assessment
   B. Diagnosis
   C. Planning
   D. Implementation
   E. Evaluation
VII. **Roles and Skills of the Home Care Nurse**
   A. Educator
   B. Advocate
   C. Psychomotor Skills
   D. Psychosocial Skills

I. Maternal and Infant Care (Straight & Harrison, 1996)

A. High-Risk Pregnancy: hyperemesis gravidarum, pregnancy-induced hypertension (PIH), placenta previa, gestational diabetes

1. In the recent past, most clients with these diagnoses were not cared for by home health agencies; care was through visits to a primary care provider, at home by family members, or in the acute care setting; more recently, with the changes managed care has brought about (see Chap. 17), these clients are followed by home health nurses at home rather than in the acute care setting

2. Treatment: depends on diagnosis; severity of the altered state of wellness; client's knowledge base; history of compliance; whether care can be safely managed at home

   3.   The nurse's role: assessment, monitoring, teaching, referrals, direct provision of care

   4.   Supplies/equipment: minimal with these diagnoses; PIH clients need a scale, urine measuring and testing supplies; diabetic clients need a glucometer and associated diabetic care supplies

   5.   Additional services: may include a home health aide, social worker, registered dietitian

   6.   Referrals: include services of WIC (Women, Infant, and Children) food supplement program, AFDC (financial aid to families with dependent children); employee benefit offices; state disability services; other diagnosis-related and personal/family services as needed

B. Postpartal Complications: related to preexisting maternal health problems (anemia, substance abuse, PIH, diabetes, emotional instability)

   1.   Most complications present symptoms and are recognized within 72 hours after delivery; ideally treatment begins in the acute care setting

   2.   With early postpartum discharge, complications may not be recognized until the client is home

   3.   Some insurers provide home health nurse visits based on specific discharge criteria (infant bonding or feeding pattern, maternal emotional state) or by diagnosis (cesarean delivery)

C. Maternal/newborn follow-up

   1.   Some insurers provide one or two home health visits after a normal uncomplicated vaginal delivery or after a planned cesarean delivery especially when the new mother experiences a short hospital stay (24 to 48 hours, vaginal delivery; 48 to 72 hours, cesarean delivery)

   2.   Home health nurses focus care on maternal and infant assessment, teaching personal and infant care, anticipatory guidance, and making referrals as needed

   3.   Related North American Nursing Diagnosis Association (NANDA) approved nursing diagnoses:

      a. Anxiety
      b. Body Image Disturbance
      c. Risk for Infection
      d. Risk for Injury
      e. Knowledge Deficit
      f. Pain
      g. Altered Parenting
      h. Altered Role Performance
      i. Self-Care Deficit
      j. Sexual Dysfunction
      k. Altered Patterns of Elimination

healthy coping strategies; instruct how to safely individualize caregiving as needed, in relation to extent of surgery, surgery site, general health or age of client

4. Trauma and injuries: goal is to assist client and family in recovering from or coping with the effects of the trauma or injury as physically and psychologically intact as possible; nursing activities are related to the nature of the injury, effect on the client and family, prognosis for full recovery, recovery with transitional limitations, or chronic limitations; effects of the trauma may be chronic with extensive rehabilitation needs; documentation and follow-up depend on nature of the trauma, effects on client and family, client and family coping skills; caregiving is a team effort with physical therapists, social workers, occupational therapists working in collaboration with home health nurses, aides, and physician

B. Chronic Illness

1. AIDS (pediatric AIDS nursing is a highly skilled area of home health nursing): goal is to promote a high quality of life within the limits of the condition; as an infectious and chronic illness with nearly a 100% mortality rate, client disease sequelae must be cared for by home health nurses skilled in pediatrics and the newest life-extending AIDS treatments, who possess the psychosocial skills needed to be effective with chronically ill and terminally ill clients; caregiving needs are broad with a strong psychosocial and holistic focus, similar to working with hospice clients; most AIDS clients' families choose to become hospice clients

2. Cancers (such as leukemia and tumors): goal is to achieve a cure; if not possible, then a lengthy remission is the goal; a nursing goal is to have the client and family be as knowledgeable and involved in the treatment choices as possible and provide them with the support needed to sustain them throughout the diagnosis and treatment process; nursing activities have a strong psychosocial focus and includes skills in chemotherapeutic agents and infusion therapies; large home health agencies in urban areas can specialize in pediatric IV therapies; because the skills are so specialized, in rural areas one or two nurses in an agency may provide the care to pediatric clients, this ensures needed specialization

3. Genetic malformations and diseases (such as congenital heart disease, cleft lip and palate, spina bifida, hemophilia): goal is to sustain life (nutrition, rest, sleep, hygiene) during diagnosis, corrective or palliative surgeries; nursing activities include emotional support and anticipatory guidance, physical caregiving

D. Infant Illness

1. Congenital malformations: cleft lip and palate, spin
   congenital heart disease (see this chapter, Section]
   Care, B. Chronic illness)
2. Newborn conditions treated at home: hyperbilir
   treated with portable phototherapy
3. Inherited diseases: phenylketonuria (PKU), cystic fi
   agnosed in infancy
4. Acquired newborn/infant conditions: systemic
   treated with intravenous (IV) antibiotics; preventab
   nicable diseases treated symptomatically, such as per
   cella, rubella, rubeola

II. Child Care

A. Acute Illness (types, goal and main nursing actions)

1. Burns: goal is to promote infection-free healing i
   time as possible; nursing actions—assess wound
   parental (caretaker) dressing change techniques
   child coping strategies; diversional activities for (
   child; primary health care provider follow-u
   needed; evaluate current therapies for goal achiev
   municate findings with physician, initiate any ch
   in response to evaluation
2. Infections: goal is to resolve current infectious pr
   vent a recurrence; infections are local (wound),
   systemic effects (pneumonia, hepatitis); system
   communicable diseases (pertussis, rubella); pro
   compliance with prescribed treatment regimen
   and/or wound care; conduct assessments for s
   toms of infection response to treatment and r
   universal infection control measures to preven
   (**handwashing,** tissue disposal, use of dispos
   safe dressing disposal of soiled supplies); comn
   effectively when documenting, contact phys
   teach new and/or reinstruct practices as ne
   family, or caretaker; suggesting age-appropria
   tivities may be part of the nurse's role; nurses
   occupational therapist, teacher, counselor as a
3. Surgeries: goal is to recover from surgery, fr
   as short a time as possible in order to retur
   wellness and activity; nursing activities incl
   ment, dressing changes if ordered, observ
   caregiver dressing change technique, teach
   age good technique; teach signs and symp
   possible complications, when to call the ph
   or parents tertiary prevention activities su
   balanced diet, adequate rest and exercise, |

and/or teaching postoperative care, initiating referrals to appropriate interprofessionals as needed to promote quality of life; evaluate caregiving against expected outcomes, modify care as needed to achieve goals, modify goals as client condition changes; document care in record appropriately, confer with physician regularly and as needed, case conference with professionals involved, client (age appropriate) and family to refine habilitative and rehabiliatative process, recognize that some inherited conditions must be managed for a lifetime and psychosocial needs change as the child ages and transitions into adulthood

4. Diabetes mellitus, type I (insulin-dependent diabetes): goal is to maintain appropriate blood glucose levels within the changing growth and activity needs of a child to prevent the detrimental effects on body systems while maintaining a high level of wellness and normal life activities as the chronic illness is managed; nursing activities include teaching, providing emotional support, monitoring, assessing client's and parent's skills in diabetic care including insulin administration; a plan of care is developed based on individual client needs; implementation follows according to the plan; evaluation is determined by the success in meeting identified outcome goals

III. Adult and Older Adult Care

A. Acute Illness: selected acute illnesses managed in home care

1. Burns: goal is to sustain life, prevent infection, and limit the effects of the burns on the client's future activities of daily living; rehabilitate client to the fullest extent possible; nursing activities and evaluation of care same as for children (see this chapter, Section I, Child Care, A. Acute Illness, 1. Burns)

{special considerations—depth of burns, amount of body surface area involved, age (very young and very old), underlying health status, and support systems—important factors affecting treatment needs and overall prognosis}

2. Infections (such as pulmonary infections [pneumonia, tuberculosis], infected wounds, infections related to infusion devices, and hepatitis): goal is to resolve the infectious status by eliminating the infection within the client; maintaining medication and treatment regimen compliance to eliminate exposure to others and improving knowledge and use of universal precautions; nursing activities are broad, depending on the type of infectious process (see this chapter, Section II, Child Care, A. Acute and B. Chronic Illness) and the psychosocial needs of individual clients

{special considerations—needs will differ depending on the type of infectious process, age (very young and very old), underlying health status, and support systems; note that 25% of AIDS clients also have tuberculosis diagnosed within the same year, universal precautions extend to body fluids *and* respiratory precautions with these clients}

3. Surgeries (such as spinal fusion, amputations, ostomies, mastectomy, and prostatectomy [there are many types of surgeries; those highlighted have significance for impact on mobility, body image, and sexuality]): goal is to experience an unremarkable postoperative period with successful adaptation to the effects on activities of daily living after the surgery; nursing activities include client assessment (overall and surgical site specific), teaching appropriate postoperative wound care to client and/or caregiver and encourage associated level of mobility recommended; encouraging tertiary prevention practices of diet, rest, exercise to place the body in the best condition for optimal recovery; prevent further bodily insult; promote coping skills; educate in new self-care practices; individualize care plans for each client; base outcomes on realistic client goals; document care appropriately; due to the complexity of changes that may occur after some surgeries, refer client to appropriate interprofessional team member

m

{special considerations—needs will differ depending on the type and invasiveness of surgery, underlying health status, and support systems; note some surgeries have physical and psychological effects on the client's sexuality; some deal with feelings of loss, frustration, adjusting to prostheses, dealing with significant others and their ability to cope, in addition to the client's own ability to cope; home health nurses need to be aware of the range of emotions, encourage expression, and refer client and significant others to appropriate resources, such as counselors, psychologists, social workers, enterostomy specialists, durable equipment companies, or prosthetic specialists}

B. Chronic Illness—selected illnesses managed in home care
  1. Alzheimer's disease and related dementias
  2. Cancers
      a. Active treatment
      b. Palliative and supportive treatment
      c. Hospice programs
  3. Heart disease
      a. Angina
      b. Myocardial infarction
      c. Arteriosclerosis (with peripheral vascular disease)
      d. Congestive heart failure
      e. Pacemaker

4. Pulmonary disease
   a. Chronic obstructive pulmonary disease (COPD)
   b. Asthma
5. Immobility/paralysis
   a. Arthritis/osteoporosis
   b. Cerebral vascular accidents (CVA)
   c. Paraplegia/quadriplegia
6. Diabetes mellitus type II (non-insulin dependent)
   a. Newly diagnosed
   b. Effects of degenerative processes
7. HIV/AIDS
   a. In-home therapies
   b. Hospice care

   {special considerations—AIDS clients typically supplement self-care with home health services as the disease progresses and treatment options become more complex; hospitalization may occur when the client begins a new treatment regimen or cannot be effectively managed at home; most AIDS clients want to be at home; issues unique to this population include decision making regarding the use of new experimental and potential life-extending treatments; death and dying issues before a "full life" is lived; leaving dependent and, at times, orphaned children; the home care nurse who serves the AIDS client needs well-developed psychosocial and technical skills}

8. Mental health disorders
   a. Depression
   b. Bipolar disorders
   c. Paranoid schizophrenia

   {special considerations—psychiatric home care nursing is relatively new and has special issues unique to the population served: safety, boundary issues, and maintaining a healthy therapeutic alliance (Daudell-Strejc & Murphy, 1995); the psychiatric home care nurse as a case manager also does the "hands-on" nursing (Quinlan & Ohlund, 1995)}

9. Neurologic conditions
   a. Parkinson's disease
   b. Multiple sclerosis (MS)
   c. Seizure disorders
10. Renal disease
    a. Glomerulonephritis, nephrosis
    b. Renal failure in clients who use various peritoneal dialysis methods

      11.   Sensory changes

          a.   Vision: glaucoma, cataracts (cataract surgery), macular degeneration

          b.   Hearing: conductive or nerve damage loss

C. **Alterations From Basic Needs: alterations in meeting basic survival needs occur with certain disease processes, trauma or injury; alterations become a concern for the home health nurse as a primary reason for making home visits or as one of the diagnoses that the nurse deals with as a part of the care provided, such as:**

      1.   Oxygenation: nasal oxygen, endotracheal oxygen, ventilator dependence (stationary or portable)

      2.   Nutrition: nasogastric feeding tubes, gastric feeding tubes, total parenteral nutrition (TPN)

      3.   Rest and sleep: patterns may be disturbed due to pain, boredom, depression, or invasive life-support equipment or treatment regimens

      4.   Elimination: transitional alterations occur in relation to medication regimen (constipation—iron supplements, inadequate fluid intake, immobility); diagnosis (diarrhea—colitis; urinary retention—paralysis); long-term or permanent alterations occur due to system failure (incontinence—indwelling catheter) or life-saving surgery (colostomy)

      5.   Safety and security: ability to remain safe may be compromised in relation to mobility alterations (post-amputation, post-CVA, altered vision, weakness) or security compromised related to altered decision-making processes (paranoid schizophrenia, Alzheimer's disease, CVA)

      6.   Mobility: client may not be mobile enough to maintain an intact integumentary system; break down of this system may be hastened by incontinence and malnutrition; safe mobility is compromised by sensory deficits, a cluttered environment, and dementia processes

D. **Nursing Diagnoses**

      1.   **Nursing diagnoses assist nurses in all settings develop nursing care plans and speak a common language when delivering care.**

      2.   Nursing diagnoses listed in some publications are grouped by diseases/disorders for easier use.

      3.   Selected nursing diagnoses have been incorporated in several chapters of this review book when discussing major diagnostic groups; for a comprehensive listing other sources must be used.

      4.   NANDA-approved nursing diagnoses are updated regularly with new diagnoses; a complete listing is available in various

nursing textbooks and editions of *Taber's Cyclopedic Medical Dictionary,* 17th ed. (Thomas, 1993)

5.   Home health agencies vary in expectations regarding the use of NANDA-approved nursing diagnoses; an agency may choose to modify them or provide a selected list used with the client diagnoses they typically served; introduction to a modified use of nursing diagnoses should be part of each new nurse's orientation to the agency

IV.   Supplies and Equipment

A.   Intravenous Equipment

1.   IV services and supplies are often offered separate from home health care agencies by infusion therapy services

2.   Nurses who specialize in IV therapy provide the setup and initiation of the service in the client's home

3.   Depending on several variables (skill level needed to administer the IV, urban or rural client location, skills of nurses in home care agencies, philosophy of physicians or agencies), the in-home caregiver, client (who has received training in the specific equipment), home health nurse, or infusion therapy nurse administers the medication, maintains the equipment, and cares for the IV at port of entry, such as changing occlusive dressings (Campbell, 1996)

4.   If the client or caregiver administers and maintains the IV, regular home visits are made by a registered nurse to assess the effectiveness of the medication, to assess the client and IV port of entry for signs and symptoms of infection, to answer questions, and to reinforce appropriate technique

B.   Equipment Distributors

1.   Local distributors (called durable medical equipment [DME] companies) deliver equipment used in the home for clients who need assistance

2.   Supplies and equiment should be ordered by hospital discharge coordinators or by the home health nurse upon completing an initial home visit and home assessment

3.   Typical equipment includes hospital beds, Hoyer lifts, commode chairs, wheelchairs, walkers, canes, and so forth

C.   Dressing Supplies

1.   Home care nurses order dressing supplies from DME companies or maintain a central supply of dressings within the agency

2.   Variety of dressing supplies are abundant; the home care arena is often on the "cutting edge" of using innovative dressing supplies; many may be new to the acute care nurse transitioning to home care

3. Often the home care nurse informs a physician of new wound care products and obtains an order to use them on the client's wound

D. Oxygen Therapy

1. In-home oxygen therapy services are often provided by companies who specialize in oxygen: tanks, concentrators, tubings and supplies
2. Paraprofessionals deliver, set up, and instruct the client and/or caregiver in the safe use of oxygen
3. Oxygen concentration in arterial blood (blood gases) is drawn at periodic intervals by registered nurses skilled in phlebotomy

V. Technology in the Home: high-tech changes are so rapid, appropriate training is needed for the staff who will use the medical device, technique, or experimental medication (Smith, 1995)

A. Pumps: to deliver patient-controlled pain medication, insulin, and antibiotics

B. Ventilators: stationary and portable units to assist client-initiated respirations or to initiate all respirations

C. Phlebotomy: home health nurses draw blood from clients for all laboratory tests ordered, including arterial blood for blood gases; this may be a new skill for an acute care nurse where laboratory staff do the phlebotomy

D. Phototherapy: use of portable home units to deliver ultraviolet light to infants with hyperbilirubinemia

E. Nutritional Supplementation: TPN, feeding tubes (nasal and gastric)

F. Elimination Technology: in-home dialysis methods, biofeedback for incontinence, indwelling catheters, suprapubic catheters, obtaining sterile urine specimens from catheters, or clean-catch urine specimens, enemas to treat elimination problems and for medication instillation as a treatment

G. New or Experimental Therapies: for specific diagnoses, such as AIDS clients and aerosol therapy; cancer clients and IV chemotherapy

VI. The Nursing Process

A. Assessment

1. Home care nurses must be skilled in assessment
2. The nurse may be the only health care professional seeing the client for weeks; it is her/his assessment and follow-up that determine the client's well-being and outcome

B. Diagnosis

1. Nursing diagnoses are disease- or disorder-related and follow the NANDA recommendations or the standards of the agency

  2. Third-party payers require that care be initiated from professional opinions that can be objectively measured; nursing diagnoses place nurses' professional opinions into a standard language

C. **Planning**

  1. The plan of care is developed by the case manager or primary nurse

  2. The plan of care provides a framework that all agency nurses follow; in most agencies, more than one nurse will provide care to a client over the period of service (because of weekends, holidays, days off, illness coverage by others)

D. **Implementation**

  1. Implementation is the action phase of the plan and is followed according to the parameters outlined in the plan

  2. Implementation continues until the evaluation phase

  3. Implementation, as planned, is discontinued if the client experiences untoward effects or is rehospitalized

  4. **Ideally, evaluation is continuous and concurrent throughout the implementation phase; changes may or may not be made at this time**

E. **Evaluation**

  1. Expected outcomes are measured; if treatment goals are not accomplished, changes may be made

  2. The client is reassessed, a new diagnosis may be made, a new plan is generated, implementation strategies begin, completing the cycle which begins again as long as service is provided

VII. **Roles and Skills of the Home Care Nurse**

A. **Educator**

  1. Clients, caregivers, paraprofessionals in the home need to be taught caregiving skills specific to the needs of the client; caregivers take over the care from home health aides when services are discontinued; in some situations, there are no caregivers and the client must have the needed skills when home health services are completed

  2. Home health nurses often teach peers; in the role of preceptor for new nurses or nursing students in the agency; to teach peers specific skills they have learned; as the agency's inservice coordinator, a full-time or part-time role, depending on the size and needs of the agency

B. **Advocate**

  1. The home care nurse may be the only professional visiting the client; it becomes her/his responsibility to speak on behalf of the client to accomplish what needs to be done

2. The advocacy role is broad and limited by the perceived role of the nurse or agency protocol and may include:
   a. Acquiring needed health care services and supplies
   b. Arranging delivery of equipment and supplies
   c. Arranging transportation for medical appointments
   d. Making supplemental health care appointments to dentist, podiatrist, and so forth
   e. Clarifying primary and consulting physician instructions
   f. Making needed referrals
   g. Intervening with landlords, utility services, and so forth
   h. Arranging for pet grooming and treatment

C. Psychomotor Skills
   1. New equipment is always being introduced in the home care arena; product manufacturers provide inservices on their new products, give discounts to agencies and clients who will use them; provide technical back-up for the use and maintenance of the equipment or product; many of the new products have computer parts and require a certain amount of psychomotor and technological skill to operate
   2. Clients coming out of the acute care setting are more acutely ill and require almost "intensive-care unit" equipment in the home; this equipment may eventually be managed by caregivers, not professionals in the home
   3. The home health nurse begins the services, establishes an in-home routine, teaches the client and caregiver(s), and may turn the caregiving over to lay caregivers before home health services are discontinued
   4. Most clients are off high-technology equipment when home care services are terminated; however, some clients are sustained indefinitely at home on life support devices, managed by paid or volunteer caregivers and family members

D. Psychosocial Skills
   1. As in community health nursing, the nurse in home health is a guest in the client's home; clients are in their domain and interact with significant others regularly; the nurse is the "outsider"
   2. Providing nursing care in a client's home puts the nurse in a position within the family system of functioning which is personal
   3. Psychosocial skills are as important as psychomotor and cognitive skills; in the acute care setting where nurses work primarily

with other professionals in an arena where the client is a guest, an individual nurse's psychosocial skills may not have as great an impact as they do in the home
4. Nurses in home care work with clients and families in crisis; this demands sensitive psychosocial skills from the nurse
5. Home care nurses work closely with a broad and diverse group of interprofessionals, paraprofessionals, and family members; each spends time consulting with the nurse; this challenges the psychosocial skills of the home care nurse more than when in the acute care setting

BIBLIOGRAPHY

Campbell, K. (1996). Intravenous nursing services: Strategies for success. *Journal of Intravenous Nursing, 19*(1), 35–37.

Daudell-Strejc, D., & Murphy, C. (1995). Emerging clinical issues in home health psychiatric nursing. *Home Healthcare Nurse, 13*(2), 17–21.

Jaffe, M. S., & Skidmore-Roth, L. (1988). *Home health nursing care plans.* St. Louis, MO: C.V. Mosby Company.

Quinlan, J., & Ohlund, G. (1995) Psychiatric home care. *Home Healthcare Nurse, 13*(4), 20–24.

Rice, R. (1996). *Home health nursing practice: Concepts and application.* St. Louis, MO: Mosby–Year Book.

Smith, G. R. (1995). The risks of using complex technology in home care. *CARING Magazine,* May, 30–34.

Spradley, B. W., & Allender, J. A. (1996). *Community health nursing: Concepts and practice.* Philadelphia: Lippincott-Raven.

Straight, B. R. & Harrison L.-O. (1996). *Maternal-newborn nursing.* Lippincott Review Series. Philadelphia: Lippincott-Raven.

Thomas, C. L. (Ed.). (1993). *Taber's cyclopedic medical dictionary.* Philadelphia: F.A. Davis Company.

STUDY QUESTIONS

1. A common prenatal high-risk situation managed at home by home health nurses occurs when there is:
   a. Braxton-Hicks contractions
   b. Pregnancy-induced hypertension
   c. A 20-lb weight gain in the pregnancy
   d. Involvement in the WIC program

2. Infants may be managed at home by home health nurses when there is:
   a. Hyperbilirubinemia
   b. A birth weight of 6 lb
   c. A poor postpartum progression
   d. An infant hydrocele

3. The single most important infection control measure that can be taught to clients and families in home care is:
   a. Disposal of soiled dressings
   b. Use of tissues
   c. Use of disposable gloves
   d. Handwashing

4. One chronic illness frequently managed by home health nurses includes:
   a. AIDS
   b. Hyperbilirubinemia
   c. Pneumonia
   d. Hernia repair

5. When caring for a client with burns on his body, special caregiving considerations need to be addressed. A most important one includes the client's:
   a. Race
   b. Weight
   c. Age
   d. Attitude

6. A new area of caregiving for home health nurses includes clients with the following diagnoses/needs:
   a. Total parenteral nutrition
   b. Psychiatric disorders
   c. Intravenous therapy
   d. Diabetes mellitus

7. The use of nursing diagnoses in home health nursing:
   a. Does not exist because they are not useful

   b. Allows nurses to speak a common language
   c. Inhibits the goals of nursing care in the home
   d. is mandatory as in the acute care setting

8. Intravenous equipment and supplies used in home health care are usually:
   a. Provided by separate agencies
   b. Reserved only for the very ill
   c. Brought to the home by the home health nurse
   d. Too expensive to use frequently

9. If a home care client needs a wheelchair, commode and a Hoyer lift, they will be delivered by a:
   a. Home health aide from the home health agency
   b. Volunteer who works with the client
   c. Durable medical equipment company
   d. Discharge planner from the hospital

10. High-tech nursing care and equipment are significant concepts for home health nurses because:
    a. They are just starting to come into the home care setting
    b. Most acute care nurses do not deal with technology
    c. They are a major and increasing part of practice
    d. Home health nurses do not deal with technology

ANSWER KEY

1. *Correct response: b*

   The alternative answer choices are normal occurrences during the prenatal period and alone do not signal a need for home health nursing services.

   Comprehension/Safe Care/Analysis

2. *Correct response: a*

   Alternative answer choices **b** and **d** are normal occurrences in newborns that alone do not signal a need for home health nursing services.

   Choice **c** may initiate home health care for the postpartum mother.

   Comprehension/Safe Care/Analysis

3. *Correct response: d*

   Handwashing is the most important infection control measure. Each of the alternative choices is important but may or may not be a part of the caregiving needs of clients, whereas correct handwashing is always a need.

   Comprehension/Safe Care/Analysis

4. *Correct response: a*

   The alternative answer choices are examples of acute conditions occurring in infants and adults. AIDS is considered chronic; people live with the diagnosis for 10 or more years.

   Comprehension/NA/Analysis

5. *Correct response: c*

   The alternative answer choices may have varying degrees of significance, but answer choice **c** has the greatest impact on recovery and prognosis.

   Application/Safe Care/Implementation

6. *Correct response: b*

   Answer choices **a** and **c** have been caregiving needs provided for 15 or more years by nurses in home health agencies. The diagnosis of diabetes mellitus is one of the oldest client diagnoses served by home health agencies.

   Application/Safe Care/Implementation

7. *Correct response: b*

   Answer choices **a, c,** and **d** are not true. Many agencies use nursing diagnoses. They do not hinder nursing care in any setting, nor is it universally mandatory that they be used.

   Application/Safe Care/Planning

8. *Correct response: a*

   The alternative answer choices are incorrect. IVs are used by all people regardless of level of overall wellness; cost of IV administration is less at home than in the acute care setting and in most agencies are not usually brought to the client's home and set up by the home health nurse.

   Application/Safe Care/Implementation

9. *Correct response: c*

   None of the people mentioned in the alternative answer choices are the appropriate people to deliver the mentioned equipment. A durable medical equipment company delivers, sets up, and at times instructs in safe use.

   Application/Safe Care/Implementation

10. *Correct response: c*

   Technology has been a part of home health nursing for 20 years or more. Both home care and acute care nurses need to be familiar with technology. Technology is increasing in home care and will continue to do so.

   Application/Safe Care/Implementation

COMPREHENSIVE EXAM—QUESTIONS

1. The World Health Organization's definition of health:
   a. States health is physical, mental, and social well-being
   b. Documents how to achieve a high level of wellness
   c. Allows for an individual adaptation to stress
   d. Focuses on the health of entire populations and communities

2. An example of primary prevention includes:
   a. Physical therapy for an arm injury
   b. Scoliosis screening among junior high-school–age children
   c. TB skin tests for agency employees
   d. Participating in a regular exercise program

3. An example of *secondary prevention* includes:
   a. Physical therapy for an arm injury
   b. Scoliosis screening among junior-high-school–age children
   c. Eating a well-balanced diet low in fat
   d. Participating in a regular exercise program

4. Community health nursing focuses primarily on:
   a. Individuals
   b. Families
   c. Groups
   d. Populations

5. A community health nurse has many roles. One of the following roles includes working with professionals from many different disciplines to provide holistic care with a wellness focus.
   a. Educator
   b. Collaborator
   c. Leader
   d. Clinician

6. Origins of public health efforts trace back to:
   a. The Bible
   b. Primitive humans
   c. Hipprocrates
   d. The Roman Empire

7. We credit the following nurse as being the first public health nurse; she also established the Henry Street Settlement in New York City.
   a. Martha Rogers
   b. Dorothea Dix
   c. Virginia Henderson
   d. Lillian Wald

8. The first occupational health nurse in the United States was Ada Stewart who worked for the:
   a. Henry Street Settlement House
   b. Metropolitan Insurance Company
   c. Vermont Marble Company
   d. Pennsylvania Railroad

9. The Frontier Nursing Service brought nursing services to people living in:
   a. The Texas panhandle
   b. Eastern Kentucky
   c. The mountains of Wyoming
   d. The American desert

10. The Pan American Health Organization (PAHO) is:
    a. A new agency started by the WHO in Central America
    b. The governing body of the WHO
    c. The oldest of the six regional offices of the WHO
    d. An organization to compete with the WHO to improve services

11. Title XVIII of the Social Security Act provided funding for health insurance for the elderly and permanently disabled. This program is called:
    a. Medicaid
    b. Medicare
    c. Supplemental Security Income
    d. Diagnostic-Related Groups

12. At the state level of health care, the services that can be expected fall in the category of:
    a. Direct—such as clinic and individual health care services

Answer sheet provided on page 295

285

b. Indirect—such as consultation and support

c. Evaluating—evaluates federal health programs

d. Planning—for the services needed in the nation

13. When writing letters to legislators, it is important to remember to:
a. Use form letters to be consistent and to promote tallying them
b. Not challenge legislators' opinions; it is viewed negatively
c. Write about negative issues; positive ones take up legislators' time
d. Express your own opinion and provide useful data familiar to you

14. Common dimensions of a community include:
a. Money, buildings, and transportation
b. Equipment, resources, and talent
c. A place, people, and social system
d. Water, land, and a source of energy

15. A nurse is exploring elder abuse issues in her community. She does a community assessment, which focuses on all factors in this community contributing to this issue. This would be called a:
a. Familiarization, orientation, or "windshield survey" assessment
b. Comprehensive assessment
c. Problem-oriented assessment
d. Subsystem assessment

16. A method of gathering data for a community assessment that includes gathering a group of interested community members to study aspects of a particular issue is an example of a(n):
a. Focus group
b. Interview
c. Community forum
d. Survey

17. Descriptors of a healthy community include:
a. A community where no members are ill or injured
b. Seeking to make its resources available to all members

c. One leader who makes the decisions for community members

d. Keeping subgroups informed of community changes when necessary

18. A working definition of *group* presented in this chapter is:
a. "Persons engaged in repeated, face-to-face communication"
b. "People who share environmental and social characteristics"
c. "A unified system of people who solve problems"
d. "Marked and unique personal characteristics"

19. A community health nurse shows a video on parenting skills to a young family. This is an example of which of the following domains of learning:
a. Psychomotor
b. Cognitive
c. Affective

20. Client readiness to learn is basic to the teaching/learning process. Which of the following factors *most* influence a client's readiness to learn?
a. The educational setting
b. Reinforcing the skills the client already has
c. Client participation in planning the class
d. Emotional and developmental level of the client

21. A method of presenting basic informative content to a group of clients can be accomplished by the following teaching method:
a. Lecture
b. Role playing
c. Demonstration
d. Discussion

22. A community health nurse is often the *case manager* for care to clients. Which of the following *best* describes essential activities to the role?
a. Listens, counsels, knows one's own limitations, and makes referrals
b. Assesses, plans, directs, controls, and evaluates the overall care

c. Teaches, promotes the public's health, works with community groups

d. Studies, collects, analyzes data, interprets results, shares the findings

23. A problem-solving board is used in the health-planning process to:

a. Design different paths or branches to choose as planning progresses

b. Provide a graphic display of alternative solutions to problems

c. Give incentives for program development in a competitive market

d. Guide people through the steps that must be taken

24. Which of the following is true about program evaluation?

a. Evaluation is an important phase of the planning process.

b. The evaluation is designed and conducted by the clients.

c. Benefits include federal government reimbursements.

d. Evaluation determines employee benefits.

25. The term *PERT* in health-program planning refers to:

a. People, Environment, Resources and Timing in the planning process

b. The administration of the overall program being developed

c. A system called Program Evaluation and Review Technique

d. A chart used to visualize the timeframe to accomplish steps in planning

26. The ultimate goal of the community health nurse's involvement in planning health programs should be to:

a. Stay very involved, preferably as a leader, throughout the process

b. Lead the project throughout the implementation phase

c. Provide some general ideas but go on about actual nursing tasks

d. Develop leadership skills in group members for community control

27. In the rural, mountainous area of Madera County, California, there are al-

ways three or four cases of plague identified in squirrels. This year, the health department has identified five cases of plague in squirrels. This change indicates that this year plague in Madera County is:

a. Systemic

b. Endemic

c. Epidemic

d. Pandemic

28. So far this winter, Willow Glen Rest Home has had 20 residents diagnosed with the flu. During the week of January 10–17, 4 cases were identified. The flu statistics for this 1 week is known as the:

a. Immunity status

b. Prevalence

c. Morbidity

d. Incidence

29. When conducting epidemiologic research, the *natural history* of a disease needs to be identified. This information includes the following:

a. The progress of the disease in the case(s) being studied

b. Determining the extent and distribution of the case(s) being studied

c. Planning a control strategy and identifying the vulnerable population

d. With all conditions present, a disease follows its pattern of development

30. The nurses in a local health department are going to conduct an epidemiologic investigation on tuberculosis in their service area. A source of data that would be most helpful to them would be:

a. Local reportable disease data

b. Census data

c. Disease registries

d. The National Center for Health Statistics (NCHS)

31. In the 1800s, positive growth of an environmental health movement in the United States was thwarted by:

a. The independent spirit of the people involved in westward movement
b. The complexities of the terrain found in the western states
c. Weather conditions not expected by the immigrants moving west
d. The religious and economic issues existing in the 1800s

32. An example of a chemical causative agent affecting the environment is:
a. Household cleaners
b. Population overcrowding
c. Toxic plants
d. The structure of office furniture

33. In the document *Healthy People 2000,* one will find:
a. US health promotion and disease prevention objectives
b. The diseases, illnesses, and accidents affecting people in the United States
c. Formulas for keeping people in the United States healthy
d. Profiles of what a healthy person in the United States looks like

34. Air pollution is a serious environmental health issue. Air pollution:
a. Is a recent phenomenon, coming about since the 1970s
b. Is the most hazardous source of biologic contamination
c. Results from industrial and automotive emissions
d. Has been a major problem since the beginning of time

35. Waste disposal in the United States is of concern because:
a. Nontoxic landfills are not satisfactory methods of handling wastes
b. The ideal disposal of wastes is to ship them to isolated places
c. Burning wastes is the only effective way of handling disposal
d. Each person in the United States produces almost two tons of waste a year

36. When solving environmental health problems, the community health nurse seeks solutions to the problem, meets with appropriate community members who decide on methods of solving the problem, and formulates an effective method of solving the problem. This is which one of the following phases of the nursing process:
a. Assessment
b. Planning
c. Implementation
d. Evaluation

37. A *theory* is defined as:
a. Disassociated and flexible ideas that add interest to a study
b. A set of systematically interrelated concepts or hypotheses
c. An idea based on intuition, not necessarily supported by data
d. A way of looking at and changing some phenomenon

38. The value of nursing theory to community health nursing includes:
a. Guiding nursing practice in the complex setting of the community
b. Viewing community problems through the eyes of community members
c. Improvement of health care access in the community
d. Eliminating barriers to conducting community studies

39. A theorist who bases a nursing theory on self-care principles is:
a. Rogers
b. Orem
c. Knowles
d. Neuman

40. A class conducted by a community health nurse who uses the Knowles Adult Learning Theory would include:
a. Objectives written by the nurse in advance of the class to save time
b. A class structure that allows for large amounts of information sharing
c. Class activities built on the students' experiences and learning needs
d. Continuous teacher evaluations to encourage achievement

41. The role of the community health nurse when working with day care and preschool centers includes:
a. Managing the center's day-to-day operation

b. Developing fund-raising opportunities to enhance resources

c. Working with center staff to assess the children's health and safety needs

d. Formulating goals that meet international safety standards

42. The role of the community health nurse in the public school system includes:

a. Identical responsibilities to the teachers and administration

b. Services focusing on providing a healthy and safe school environment

c. Disciplining children not complying with immunization guidelines

d. Planning and implementing the educational curriculum

43. Ergonomic factors in the work setting affect the employee and include the:

a. Equipment designs in the workplace

b. Fiscal management of the company

c. Ethnic and racial mix of the workers

d. Size and location of the company

44. Stressors that are unique to the agricultural work setting include:

a. Boredom with repetitive activities and noise pollution

b. Exposure to toxic substances and physical demands

c. Long meetings, deadlines, and conflict with managers

d. Sitting for long hours and prolonged periods of inactivity

45. A congregate living setting can be identified by the following characteristics:

a. A building made of concrete and stone with limited wood products

b. Private living quarters with group dining and some social services

c. A residence inhabited by a family with one or more members

d. Residents who depend on regular skilled nursing services.

46. When working with the incarcerated, there is *one* major difference from other community settings that nurses work in:

a. The clients are physically and verbally abusive

b. The population is ambulatory and basically well

c. Security of the population is the first priority

d. The clients do not want health care services

47. The International Nursing Honor Society, Sigma Theta Tau, has a mission to:

a. Serve as the site for national data on nursing

b. Promote excellence in nursing

c. Conduct nursing research

d. Help the nursing profession focus its direction

48. Which of the following research studies represents quantitative research?

a. Comparing the weight of children with their height

b. Determining what men perceive as their greatest health risk

c. Observing the bedtime routines of 4-year-old children

d. Inquiring about the infant bathing practices used by new mothers

49. Which of the following research studies represents qualitative research?

a. Comparing weights of infants with amount and brand of formula taken

b. Determining the number of health care provider visits made by men

c. Analyzing a group of teens' social behaviors with the opposite sex

d. Observing women for the kinds of safety practices used with children

50. Which one of the following gives an example of an experimental research study?

a. A CHN interviews parents bringing children to an immunization clinic

b. A CHN has families complete a survey on home visits made this week

c. A CHN reviews charts of office visits made by 2- and 3-year-old children last May

d. Two CHNs begin providing different services from the rest of the staff and results are measured

51. The best definition of *culture* is:

a. A biologically identified group of people who have common features

b. A group of people with common origins and a shared identity

c. The beliefs, values, and behavior that are shared as a group

d. The multiple differences in people coexisting in a location

52. Ethnocentrism in community health nursing is:

a. A desirable trait to be achieved by new community health nurses

b. An approach to clients that improves nurse–client communication

c. Positive feelings about one's culture; negative feelings about others

d. An effective way of working with culturally diverse groups of people

53. The culture and/or characteristics of Asian Americans include:

a. Different languages, values, and customs

b. Individual effort is valued over cooperation

c. Japanese is a primary language

d. Respecting children more than elders

54. Incorporating transcultural nursing concepts with the evaluation phase of the nursing process includes:

a. Gathering data about cultural values and attitudes

b. Pacing the timing of activities according to cultural group norms

c. Determining if the cultural group's goals have been achieved

d. Collaborating with the cultural community members

55. Common aspects of all definitions of a family include the following:

a. Two married people with or without children

b. Individuals sharing a residence with emotional bonds

c. People related through marriage, no matter where they live

d. A single person who lives alone with no significant others

56. Which of the following family structures represents a traditional family?

a. Homosexual couple

b. Multigenerational family

c. Cohabitating couple

d. Commune family

57. Conducting a family assessment is essential to beginning a relationship with a family. The community health nurse:

a. Focuses attention on the most dysfunctional family member

b. Asks closed-ended questions to get precise information

c. Focuses on data gathered from the head of the household

d. Collects data over several visits from all members of the family

58. The community health nurse may ask a family to diagram themselves in relation to others in their life, with strong and weak lines connecting them with others, in order to display emotional connectedness. This is called a(n):

a. Eco-map

b. Genogram

c. Social support network

d. Gantt chart

59. A healthy family includes the following characteristic:

a. Unstructured role relationships

b. Keeping distant from the broader community

c. Coping with problems by avoiding them

d. Enhancing the development of the individual

60. *Healthy People 2000* is a(n):

a. Interactive video on healthy aging in the 21st century

b. Improvement program for people in Third World countries

c. Government document with health goals for Americans in the 1990s

d. New way of looking at the health of people, through their own eyes

61. A specific need of the maternal aged (15 to 45) population in the United States is:

a. Postponing pregnancy until at least age 20

b. Deciding when pregnancy occurs, if sexually active

c. Eliminating pregnancies after age 40 due to being high risk

d. Making sure there are acute care facilities available for childbirth

62. An example of *secondary* prevention with the maternal–infant population includes:

a. Diagnosing problem pregnancies early in order to begin treatment

b. Encouraging proper diet, rest, exercise, and regular prenatal care

c. Following health practitioner recommendations for preventing illness

d. Preventing infections from occurring after a cesarean delivery

63. An example of *tertiary* prevention with the adult population is:

a. Early diagnosis and treatment of chronic illnesses, such as diabetes

b. Teaching healthy living habits to keep illnesses from occurring

c. Providing adults with skills to be effective health care consumers

d. Attempt to reduce the extent and severity of injuries that have occurred

64. Selected goals of *Healthy People 2000* for older adults include reducing:

a. Suicides among older African-American men

b. Deaths from gonorrhea

c. Epidemic pneumonia and flu deaths

d. The percentage of older adults in the United States.

65. The community health nurse's role as case manager with older adults focuses on:

a. Monitoring and evaluating older adult responses to services

b. Speaking on behalf of older adults to improve care they receive

c. Focusing on wellness when providing care to older adults

d. Cooperating with others to promote the health of elders

66. Which of the following groups of homeless is increasing in the United States?

a. Older women

b. Women with children

c. Teenagers

d. Middle-age singles

67. Substance abuse in the United States is characterized by:

a. 3 million people dependent on or abusing alcohol

b. Difficulty in acquiring prescription and illegal drugs

c. Inexpensive rehabilitation programs that are successful

d. Family disruption, violence, and crime

68. An example of tertiary prevention when working with the mentally ill population is:

a. In-patient treatment

b. Crisis intervention

c. Alternative housing placements

d. Definitive medical care

69. Preventing developmental and physical disabilities at the secondary level includes the following activities:

a. Abstaining from drugs and alcohol during pregnancy

b. Early recognition of the signs and symptoms of disability

c. Rehabilitative and long-term outpatient follow-up

d. Early and continuous routine prenatal care

70. Violence directed toward neighborhood individuals or groups, committed as an aggressive act in support of territory or as retribution for a similar attack, is characteristic of:

a. Terrorist behavior

b. Random violence

c. Gang activity

d. Domestic violence

71. A community health nurse goes to a part of town expected to be affected by a flooding creek and sets up a shelter in anticipation of many homeless families for several days. She stocks the shelter with first-aid supplies and over-the-counter medications. This is an example of what type of disaster, what level of disaster prevention and level of illness prevention:

a. Manmade; primary disaster prevention; secondary illness prevention

b. Natural; secondary disaster prevention; secondary illness prevention

c. Natural; primary disaster prevention; primary illness prevention

d. Manmade; tertiary disaster prevention; secondary illness prevention

72. A nonhuman entity that actively carries disease organisms that have the potential to infect humans is a(n):
    a. Antibody
    b. Vector
    c. Vaccine
    d. Antagonist

73. An example of secondary prevention in communicable disease control is:
    a. Administering immunizations
    b. Eliminating the infectious agent
    c. Providing long-term follow-up
    d. Screening for disease

74. According to the CDC in 1994 the one reportable communicable disease with the largest numbers in the United States was:
    a. Gonorrhea
    b. Varicella
    c. Herpes
    d. Syphilis

75. Food-borne diseases can escalate into situations with severe consequences; preventing food-borne diseases at the primary level of prevention includes:
    a. Replacing lost fluids
    b. Providing appropriate antibiotic therapy
    c. Providing supportive care
    d. Cooking meat products thoroughly

76. Tuberculosis is a disease that is:
    a. Under control and rarely seen in the community
    b. Resurging and a major community health problem
    c. Occurring mainly in the AIDS population
    d. Treated in adults but not in children

77. A client with tuberculosis, classification III, is considered to have:
    a. An infection, negative chest x-ray, but has a history of exposure
    b. No history of exposure, negative skin test, no further tests
    c. A disease, with a positive chest x-ray and sputum

d. History of exposure, negative skin test, with no further tests

78. Home health nursing is a discipline of nursing that is:
    a. Growing steadily and hires a small number of nurses
    b. A minor part of the health care system causing a minimal effect
    c. Growing fast and recruits significant numbers of nurses
    d. A declining area of nursing with a decreasing focus

79. Lillian Wald is remembered for:
    a. Developing public health and home health nursing
    b. Improving hospital nursing and medical care
    c. Formalizing the educational preparation for nurses
    d. Including community health content in nursing schools

80. Medicare influenced the home care movement by:
    a. Reimbursing clients for the cost of all care received at home
    b. Requiring physicians to direct home care and determine eligibility
    c. Broadening home care services through its reimbursement system
    d. Having a payment system to provide unique coverage in each state

81. Medicaid influences the home health services provided to clients by:
    a. Providing home health care to medically indigent clients
    b. Providing employer incentives for hiring people in poverty
    c. Aiding poor families to help themselves instead of using Medicare
    d. Combining federal, state, and local programs for the wealthy

82. Managed care is best defined as a(n):
    a. Pattern of delivering care to clients that saves driving time
    b. Efficient system of care to decrease the number of nurses needed
    c. Planning and delivery approach to care that controls quality and cost
    d. Nurse's way of managing time and resources to provide quality care

83. Different governance models exist in home health; the one that is associated with an acute care setting and is usually not for profit is a:
  a. Combination agency
  b. Proprietary agency
  c. Hospital-based agency
  d. Official agency

84. All home health care services are directed by the:
  a. Discharge planner
  b. Physician
  c. Case manager
  d. Agency administrator

85. A physical therapist is a professional staff member in a home health agency who can assist with successful client recovery goals by:
  a. Making shared visits with the nurse to assist in personal caregiving
  b. Developing and implementing individualized client rehabilitation plans
  c. Consulting with skilled nursing facilities and acute care centers
  d. Supervising care given by nurses delivering care in the home

86. Differences exist between home health nursing and nursing in the acute care setting. Which of the following is one of the differences?
  a. Physical assessment skills are not used; the clients are not as ill
  b. Nursing care is not needed in homes as much as in acute care settings
  c. Decision-making skills are not as important as in the hospital
  d. Community resource and insurance coverage information are necessary

87. Differences in home health nursing from nursing in public health agencies include:
  a. Public health nurses focus on secondary prevention and provide physical nursing care
  b. The home health population is a healthy population and not ill as in public health nursing
  c. Home health clients are older and usually more ill than clients in public health settings

  d. High-risk pregnant women, infants, and children make up most of the home health nursing caseload

88. A physician writes an order for one of your home health clients. The prescription suggests a daily dose of medication that is two times higher than the upper daily limits of that medication according to the most recent edition of a nurses' drug manual. Your best action would be to:
  a. Teach the client side effects to look for and instruct to discontinue the medication if any side effects occur
  b. Check with other nurses in the agency to see if this is a typical practice of this physician
  c. Withhold the medication from the client until clarified with the ordering physician
  d. Recommend that the client, family members, or caregiver check the order with the physician

89. You are making a home visit to Joseph Irwin, an 82-year-old man with early Alzheimer's disease. You find him on the bedroom floor with the caretaker attempting to assist him to standing with the help of a neighbor. You provide appropriate assistance, assessment, and follow-up to his physician. However, you also write up an incident report. This document objectively states what you observed and actions taken. The document is:
  a. An official part of the client's chart
  b. A legal document to be reserved for the client's lawyer
  c. Kept in the agency to be used for quality and risk management
  d. Documented in the client's chart that the incident report was filed

90. Some home health agencies are becoming *specialized,* which means that the agency is:
  a. Cutting back on personnel to save money
  b. Integrating levels of care and types of services

  c. Providing a few selected services
  d. Selecting one particular service to provide

91. Medicare finances home care services with the following specifications:
  a. Services designed especially for low-income elders
  b. Care is on an intermittent and part-time basis
  c. Caregiving when physician care is not needed
  d. Only when clients need the services of a social worker

92. Mountain Home Health Agency is a small agency in the rural part of Colorado. Two nurses work for the agency and care for clients miles apart. The organizational pattern of service that would provide the best care and be cost-effective is:
  a. Geographic distribution
  b. Client diagnosis
  c. Caregiver specialty
  d. Physician location

93. Central Medical Services is an urban home health agency. Many highly skilled nurses are employed with this excellent home health agency, which serves over 300 high-tech need clients in addition to 50 hospice clients. This agency may be in the best position to use which of the following organizational patterns?
  a. Geographic distribution
  b. Client location
  c. Caregiver specialty
  d. Location of physicians

94. The goal of a quality management program in a home health agency is:
  a. Skilled nursing care; it is a major part of the services provided
  b. Client satisfaction; clients know if they get good care
  c. Achieved client outcomes; this is the purpose of the caregiving
  d. High employee morale; it is a key indicator of a quality agency

95. Common high-risk prenatal situations managed at home by home health nurses include:

  a. Signs of quickening
  b. Placenta previa
  c. Weight gain between 20 and 25 lb
  d. WIC program membership

96. The most important infection control measure that can be carried out by nurses in home care is:
  a. Proper disposal of soiled dressings
  b. Use of disposable tissues instead of handkerchiefs
  c. Use of disposable gloves with clients
  d. Proper and frequent handwashing

97. A new area of caregiving for home health nurses includes clients with the following conditions:
  a. Terminal illnesses
  b. Psychiatric disorders
  c. Pregnancy-induced hypertension
  d. Diabetes mellitus

98. Nursing diagnoses are used in home health nursing:
  a. Rarely, because they are not useful in this setting
  b. And provide nurses with a common language
  c. Sparingly, because it inhibits the nursing goals
  d. Because it is mandatory to use them

99. If a home care client needs a hospital bed, wheelchair, and a cane, they will be delivered by a(n):
  a. Agency home health aide
  b. Hospital or home health agency volunteer
  c. Durable medical equipment company
  d. Home care coordinator

100. High-tech nursing care and equipment are significant for home health agencies because:
  a. High-tech care is just starting to come into home care
  b. Home health nurses do not want to deliver high-tech care
  c. It is a major and increasing part of their services
  d. Agencies have not dealt with high-tech care until recently

Answer Sheet for Comprehensive Exam

With a pencil, blacken the circle under the option you have chosen for your correct answer.

	A	B	C	D		A	B	C	D		A	B	C	D
1.	○	○	○	○	21.	○	○	○	○	41.	○	○	○	○
2.	○	○	○	○	22.	○	○	○	○	42.	○	○	○	○
3.	○	○	○	○	23.	○	○	○	○	43.	○	○	○	○
4.	○	○	○	○	24.	○	○	○	○	44.	○	○	○	○
5.	○	○	○	○	25.	○	○	○	○	45.	○	○	○	○
6.	○	○	○	○	26.	○	○	○	○	46.	○	○	○	○
7.	○	○	○	○	27.	○	○	○	○	47.	○	○	○	○
8.	○	○	○	○	28.	○	○	○	○	48.	○	○	○	○
9.	○	○	○	○	29.	○	○	○	○	49.	○	○	○	○
10.	○	○	○	○	30.	○	○	○	○	50.	○	○	○	○
11.	○	○	○	○	31.	○	○	○	○	51.	○	○	○	○
12.	○	○	○	○	32.	○	○	○	○	52.	○	○	○	○
13.	○	○	○	○	33.	○	○	○	○	53.	○	○	○	○
14.	○	○	○	○	34.	○	○	○	○	54.	○	○	○	○
15.	○	○	○	○	35.	○	○	○	○	55.	○	○	○	○
16.	○	○	○	○	36.	○	○	○	○	56.	○	○	○	○
17.	○	○	○	○	37.	○	○	○	○	57.	○	○	○	○
18.	○	○	○	○	38.	○	○	○	○	58.	○	○	○	○
19.	○	○	○	○	39.	○	○	○	○	59.	○	○	○	○
20.	○	○	○	○	40.	○	○	○	○	60.	○	○	○	○

	A	B	C	D		A	B	C	D		A	B	C	D
61.	○	○	○	○	75.	○	○	○	○	88.	○	○	○	○
62.	○	○	○	○	76.	○	○	○	○	89.	○	○	○	○
63.	○	○	○	○	77.	○	○	○	○	90.	○	○	○	○
64.	○	○	○	○	78.	○	○	○	○	91.	○	○	○	○
65.	○	○	○	○	79.	○	○	○	○	92.	○	○	○	○
66.	○	○	○	○	80.	○	○	○	○	93.	○	○	○	○
67.	○	○	○	○	81.	○	○	○	○	94.	○	○	○	○
68.	○	○	○	○	82.	○	○	○	○	95.	○	○	○	○
69.	○	○	○	○	83.	○	○	○	○	96.	○	○	○	○
70.	○	○	○	○	84.	○	○	○	○	97.	○	○	○	○
71.	○	○	○	○	85.	○	○	○	○	98.	○	○	○	○
72.	○	○	○	○	86.	○	○	○	○	99.	○	○	○	○
73.	○	○	○	○	87.	○	○	○	○	100.	○	○	○	○
74.	○	○	○	○										

COMPREHENSIVE EXAM—ANSWER KEY

1. **Correct response: a**
   Answer choices **b, c,** and **d** do not represent the focus of the WHO definition.
   Knowledge/NA/NA

2. **Correct response: d**
   a. Is an example of tertiary prevention
   b. Is an example of secondary prevention
   c. Is an example of secondary prevention
   Comprehension/Health Promotion/Implementation

3. **Correct response: b**
   a. Is an example of tertiary prevention
   c. Is an example of primary prevention
   d. Is an example of primary prevention
   Comprehension/Health Promotion/Implementation

4. **Correct response: d**
   Answers **a, b,** and **c** are served, but the focus is on the health of large groups or populations that make up communities. Elevating the health of populations elevates the health of individuals.
   Knowledge/NA/NA

5. **Correct response: b**
   a. The educator role focuses on health teaching.
   c. The leader role focuses on directing, influencing or persuading others.
   d. In the clinician role, the CHN uses nursing skills to provide a holistic focus of caregiving in a variety of ways.
   Application/NA/NA

6. **Correct response: b**
   The earliest public health efforts are documented among primitive humans. The responses in answer choices **a, c,** and **d** occurred later. Each era contributed practices that have improved public health efforts.
   Comprehension/NA/NA

7. **Correct response: d**
   a. Martha Rogers was a contemporary nurse researcher and theorist who died in the 1990s.
   b. Dorothea Dix was a teacher who committed her life to prison and mental health reform.
   c. Virginia Henderson was a contemporary nurse educator and author who died in the 1990s; the Sigma Theta Tau International nursing honor society has its library named for Ms. Henderson.
   Comprehension/NA/NA

8. **Correct response: c**
   Answer choice **a** was the community center started by Lillian Wald in 1893 for immigrant families in New York City.
   Answer choice **b** was the insurance company that started a home nursing service to its policy holders early in the 1900s, but not occupational nursing services.
   Answer choice **d** is the name of a railroad that existed before AMTRAK. It did not have the first occupational nursing services.
   Comprehension/NA/NA

9. **Correct response: b**
   Answer choices **a, c.,** and **d** are locations needing public health services, but are not the areas served by the Frontier Nursing Service.
   Comprehension/NA/NA

10. **Correct response: c**
    a. The PAHO is the oldest (1902) regional office of the WHO and provides health care services to all of the Americas and Canada, not just Central America.
    b. The WHO is the the governing body of the six regional offices; PAHO is one of the six offices.

d. It is a part of WHO, not a competing organization.

Comprehension/NA/NA

11. **Correct response: b**
    a. This is Title XIX of the Social Security Act and provides health care to people meeting low income guidelines, regardless of age.
    c. This program provides income to the poor, disabled and blind.
    d. This is a way of paying for health care, part of a prospective payment system.

Comprehension/NA/NA

12. **Correct response: b**
    a. This describes the services offered by the local level of government.
    c. This describes one of the services offered by the federal level of government.
    d. Planning is another important service of the federal level of government.

Comprehension/NA/Assessment

13. **Correct response: d**
    a. Form letters are not recommended; legislators tend not to read them.
    b. Personal opinion is desired and is the purpose of writing.
    c. Negative and positive comments are welcomed and are needed to sway a legislator's opinion.

Comprehension/NA/Analysis

14. **Correct response: c**
    Choices **a, b,** or **d** included components of each dimension. The correct response includes all the components needed for community.

Comprehension/NA/Analysis

15. **Correct response: c.** The nurse will explore all factors that contribute to the elder abuse issue, and conducts a problem-oriented assessment. The problem is elder abuse; the assessment is problem-oriented.
    Answer choices **a, b,** and **d** describe other types of community assessment.

Application/NA/Assessment

16. **Correct response: a.** This describes a focus group. This gives the nurse new data from community "experts" to add to other information as data are being gathered.
    Answer choices **b, c,** and **d** describe other methods of data collection.

Application/NA/Assessment

17. **Correct response: b.** This is one of ten descriptors shared in this chapter. It is important for the community system and its resources to be available to all community members.
    Answer choices **a, c,** and **d** describe inappropriate or unhealthy community patterns.

Application/Health Promotion/ Assessment

18. **Correct response: a**
    Answer choices **b, c,** and **d** are not a part of the definition of *group.*

Comprehension/NA/NA

19. **Correct response: b**
    Answer choice **a** pertains to eye and hand coordination skills.
    Answer choice **c** involves the emotion, feeling, or affect.

Application/Safe Care/Implementation

20. **Correct response: d**
    Answer choices **a, b,** and **c** are additional components of teaching/learning principles, just as client readiness is one of the principles. Client readiness is determined by emotional readiness, educational background, and developmental level.

Comprehension/Health Promotion/ Assessment

21. **Correct response: a**
    b. Role play—involves having clients assume and act out roles, again not a technique suited for large groups when transmitting general information
    c. Demonstration—best conducted with individuals or in small groups

with time for the participants to return a demonstration

d. Discussion—encourages two-way communication, difficult to do in a large group, and not recommended when general information is being shared

Application/Health Promotion/ Implementation

22. *Correct response: b*

Answer choice **a** describes the counselor role.

Answer choice **c** describes the teacher role.

Answer choice **d** describes the researcher role.

Comprehension/NA/Implementation

23. *Correct response: b*

Answer choice **a** describes a problem-solving board. Choices **c** and **d** do not describe any phases or tools used in health program planning.

Comprehension/NA/Planning

24. *Correct response: a*

In answer choice **b**, the clients may participate in the program evaluation by completing a survey, but they do not design or conduct program evaluations.

Answer choice **c** indicates there will be a refund of money from the government. Evaluations do not accomplish this.

Answer choice **d** is a part of the employee employment package and may be renegotiated with management but not as an outcome of an evaluation of the program itself.

Comprehension/NA/Planning

25. *Correct response: c*

Answer choices **a** and **b** do not pertain to PERT.

Answer choice **d** describes the Gantt chart used in program planning.

Comprehension/NA/Planning

26. *Correct response: d*

The remaining answer choices are wrong. They represent what is *not* desired. The nurse should not maintain

the leadership role throughout the planning or implementation, nor does the nurse just share ideas. Throughout the planning, the nurse works to create leadership skills among the health planning group members.

Application/NA/Implementation

27. *Correct response: b*

Endemic—which means that the number is relatively stable and similar to the normal or expected frequency in a community or region. Answer choices **a, c,** and **d** have different definitions not supported by this question.

Comprehension/Safe Care/Assessment

28. *Correct response: d.* The statistics from this 1 week is the incidence.

Answer choice **b** is the prevalence—the accumulated data of the flu in this institution during the winter.

Answers **a** and **c** are terms in epidemiology but not related to this situation.

Analysis/Physiologic/Analysis

29. *Correct response: d*

Answer choice **a** describes the Chain of Causation.

Answer choices **b** and **c** are the second and third steps of the epidemiologic process; determining the natural history of a disease is the first step.

Comprehension/Health Promotion/ Analysis

30. *Correct response: a.* The nurses can get specific information about this reportable disease in their community.

The other answer choices are good resources for information needed when conducting epidemiologic investigations. Census data may be helpful to give all nurses background information for any type of study. It will give information about the population as a whole—age, sex, race, housing, and so forth. Disease registries select specific diseases to focus on, and tuberculosis may not be one of them. The NCHS will have information on studies they

have conducted, and, if they have something on tuberculosis, this may be helpful. The most helpful is the statistics on locally reportable diseases.
Application/Safe Care/Implementation

31. *Correct response: a*
Situations in the remaining answer choices may have existed in the 1800s, but the situations depicted in answer **a** affected the environmental health movement more significantly.
Analysis/Health Promotion/Analysis

32. *Correct response: a*
The other answer choices are examples of psychological, biologic, and ergonomic factors, respectively.
Comprehension/Safe Care/Assessment

33. *Correct response: a*
The remaining answer choices are incorrect. *Healthy People 2000* identifies objectives we should achieve by the year 2000 in major disease and injury areas affecting people in the United States. It gives the numbers of occurrences during key years in the 1980s and projects acceptable numbers of occurrences by the year 2000.
Comprehension/Health Promotion/Assessment

34. *Correct response: c*
Answer choice **a** is incorrect. Air pollution has been a major problem since industrialization.
     Answer choice **b** is incorrect. Air pollution is hazardous due to chemical contamination.
     Answer choice **d** is incorrect because it was not a major problem until the Industrial Age. However, smoke-filled caves could have polluted the air cave dwellers inhaled.
Comprehension/Safe Care/Analysis

35. *Correct response: d*
Answer choice **a** is incorrect. A landfill is a satisfactory method of handling solid nontoxic wastes.
     Answer choice **b** is incorrect. Hiding solid waste does not solve the problem; it creates problems in another area.

Answer choice **c** is incorrect. Burning solid waste transforms it into another pollutant.
Comprehension/Safe Care/Analysis

36. *Correct response: b*
The example is from the second phase of the nursing process, planning. The other answer choices are incorrect.
Comprehension/NA/NA

37. *Correct response: b*
Answer choices **a, c,** and **d** do not correctly define a theory. Ideas are associated with and based on experiences that are supported by data, and theories describe but do not change a phenomenon.
Comprehension/NA/NA

38. *Correct response: a*
Answer choices **b, c,** and **d** do not depict the value of a nursing theory to community health nursing practice.
Comprehension/NA/NA

39. *Correct response: b*
Answer choices **a, c,** and **d** are theorists associated with the science of unitary human beings, adult learning theory, and a systems theory.
Knowledge/NA/NA

40. *Correct response: c*
Answer choices **a, b,** and **d** do not describe the use of adult learning theory. In adult learning theory, objectives would be written with the students, class structure would reflect the student's needs, and the teacher may give continuous feedback but not evaluation.
Analysis/Effective Care Environment/Evaluation

41. *Correct response: c*
Answer choices **a** and **b** are roles of the administration and staff.
     Answer choice **d** is incorrect. There are no international safety standards.
Application/NA/Implementation

42. *Correct response: b*
Answer choices **a** and **d** describe roles of teachers and administrators.

Answer choice **c** is incorrect. Children are not disciplined for not having immunizations. They may be excluded from school until parents comply with immunization standards set by the school.
Application/Safe Care/Implementation

43. *Correct response: a*
Answer choices **b, c,** and **d** are not related to the ergonomic factors of the work setting.
Application/Safe Care/Implementation

44. *Correct response: b*
Answer choice **a** describes an industrial setting.
Answer choices **c** and **d** better describe the business setting.
Analysis/Safe Care/Implementation

45. *Correct response: b*
Answer choice **a** describes the physical characteristics of a certain type of structure.
Answer choice **c** describes a private home.
Answer choice **d** describes a skilled nursing facility.
Application/NA/Analysis

46. *Correct response: c*
Answer choices **a, b,** and **d** may apply to any setting. In prisons and jails, the purpose of the facility is security. Health needs, no matter how severe, are secondary.
Application/Safe Care/Analysis

47. *Correct response: b*
Answer choices **a, c,** and **d** are incorrect.
Comprehension/NA/Analysis

48. *Correct response: a*
Answer choices **b, c,** and **d** describe samples of qualitative research where the meaning of experiences to individuals are described and studies tend to be more holistic in an attempt to understand a problem or phenomenon.
Application/NA/Implementation

49. *Correct response: c*
Answer choices **a, b,** and **d** are ex-

amples of quantitative research. Participants self-report on issues in question, behaviors are captured and counted via observation, or there is measurement of physiologic function.
Application/NA/Implementation

50. *Correct response: d*
Answer choices **a, b,** and **c** are examples of prospective and retrospective studies.
Application/NA/Implementation

51. *Correct response: c*
Answer choice **a** is the definition of *race*.
Answer choice **b** is the definition of *ethnic group*.
Answer choice **d** is the definition of *cultural diversity*.
Knowledge/NA/Assessment

52. *Correct response: c*
Answer choices **a, b,** and **d** are incorrect. Being ethnocentric is not a desirable state. Approaching clients with ethnocentric attitudes does not improve their level of wellness, and is not an effective way to deal with others.
Application/Psychosocial/Analysis

53. *Correct response: a*
Asian Americans value cooperation over competition, have many native languages that remain primary in immigrant groups, and respect elders.
Comprehension/Safe Care/Analysis

54. *Correct response: c*
Answer choice **a** is from the assessment phase, **b** is the implementation phase, and **d** is from the planning phase; each demonstrates transcultural nursing principles.
Application/Safe Care/Evaluation

55. *Correct response: b*
Answer choice **a** assumes one must be married to be considered a family; choice **c** implies a family needs to be related by bloodlines; and in choice **d** the person meets none of the characteristics of a family, as included in answer choice **b**.
Comprehension/Psychosocial/Analysis

56. *Correct response: b*
Answer choices **a**, **c**, and **d** represent new family structures that have been nontraditional in the United States.
Knowledge/NA/Assessment

57. *Correct response: d*
Answer choice **a** indicates there is a dysfunctional family member in the household; visits may be made to healthy families.
Choice **b**—questions should be open-ended and goal directed.
Choice **c**—data need to be gathered from all family members, not just the head of the household.
Application/Safe Care/Implementation

58. *Correct response: c*
Answer choices **a** and **b** are other assessment methods.
Choice **d** is a time-line chart used in planning within agencies (see Chap. 6).
Comprehension/Safe Care/Analysis

59. *Correct response: d*
Answer choice **a**—in healthy families, role relationships are structured effectively.
In choice **b**, the healthy family actively attempts to cope with problems.
In choice **c**, the healthy family establishes regular links with the broader community.
Comprehension/Safe Care/Assessment

60. *Correct response: c*
Answer choices **a**, **b**, and **d** are incorrect responses.
Comprehension/Safe Care/Assessment

61. *Correct response: b*
Answer choices **a** and **c** suggest specific ages for pregnancy and this is inappropriate. Individuals are different, and no one age is right for all people.
Answer choice **d** implies there are inadequate facilities for infant delivery. This is not a major problem in the United States. Most people live within reasonable distances from facilities with maternity services.
Application/Safe Care/Planning

62. *Correct response: a*
Answers **b** and **c** are examples of primary prevention.
Answer choice **d** is an example of tertiary prevention.
Application/Safe Care/Implementation

63. *Correct choice: d*
Answer choice **a** is an example of secondary prevention.
Answer choices **b** and **c** are examples of primary prevention.
Application/Health Promotion/Implementation

64. *Correct choice: c*
Answer choices **a**, **b**, and **d** are incorrect. None of them are goals of *Healthy People 2000*.
Application/Health Promotion/Implementation

65. *Correct response: a*
Answer choice **b** is an example of the advocate role.
Choice **c** is an example of the clinician role.
Choice **d** is an example of the collaborator role.
Application/Health Promotion/Implementation

66. *Correct response: b*
Other groups are homeless in great numbers, but women with children were not a traditional homeless population and their numbers are increasing.
Comprehension/NA/Assessment

67. *Correct response: d*
Answer choice **a** is incorrect. The number is 13 million.
Answer choice **b** is incorrect. Unfortunately, prescription and illegal drugs are readily available.
Answer choice **c**—rehabilitative programs are expensive, and the programs are often unsuccessful and repeated, which is a major problem.
Comprehension/Health Promotion/Analysis

68. *Correct response: c*
Answer choices **a, b,** and **d** are examples of secondary prevention services.
Application/Health Promotion/Implementation

69. *Correct response: b*
Answer choices **a** and **d** are examples of primary prevention.
Answer choice **c** is an example of tertiary prevention.
Application/Health Promotion/Implementation

70. *Correct response: c*
Answer choices **a, b,** and **d** describe other categories of violence present in society.
Comprehension/Psychosocial/Analysis

71. *Correct response: b*
This is a natural disaster, a natural phenomenon. The community health nurse is attempting to eliminate an additional problem caused by the flood by protecting the vulnerable community members, a goal in seconary prevention during a disaster. The nurse is not preventing the illness or injury but, with appropriate supplies, is treating them at the secondary level.
Analysis/Safe Care/Implementation

72. *Correct response: b*
Answer choices **a, c,** and **d** are incorrect responses.
Knowledge/NA/NA

73. *Correct response: d*
Answer choices **a** and **b** are examples of primary prevention.
Answer choice **c** is an example of tertiary prevention.
Analysis/Health Promotion/Implementation

74. *Correct response: a*
There were 388,000 cases of gonorrhea reported, making it the most frequently reported communicable disease. The other diseases do not have cases reported into the hundreds of thousands.
Comprehension/Physiologic/Analysis

75. *Correct response: d*
Answer choices **a** and **b** are examples of secondary prevention.
Answer choice **c** is an example of tertiary prevention.
Analysis/Health Promotion/Implementation

76. *Correct response: b*
TB is not under control. It is resurging, especially among immigrant and refugee populations, homeless, aged, infants, and among those with AIDS, and is a major community health problem. TB is treated in children and adults.
Analysis/Safe Care/Planning

77. *Correct response: c*
Tuberculosis, classification III, is considered TB disease. Classification II is considered an infection, must have a history of exposure, positive skin test, but chest x-ray is negative. TB is not considered an infection unless there is a positive skin test.
Answer choices **a** and **d** are TB, classification I.
Answer choice **b** is TB, classification 0.
Analysis/Health Promotion/Implementation

78. *Correct response: c*
The other choices do not accurately reflect home health nursing as it is today.
Comprehension/NA/NA

79. *Correct response: a*
Lillian Wald did not work to alter nursing or medical care delivered in hospitals. She did not change the educational requirements of new graduates or the curriculum of nursing schools. Nursing graduates at the turn of the century were hired to work in family's homes, caring for the ill, after training in hospitals. That was the norm.
Comprehension/NA/NA

80. *Correct response: b*
In answer choice **a**, Medicare does not cover all the needs of clients. Guidelines are very specific as to what is covered.

Answer choice **c** suggests Medicare has broadened the definition of home care. It has actually narrowed it to a medical-based model of service.

Answer choice **d** indicates Medicare is a state system. It is a federal system with care reimbursed in the same way in each state. Medicaid is a system unique in each state.

Comprehension/NA/Analysis

81. *Correct response: a*
Medicaid supplements Medicare or is the primary payer for the medically indigent. It is a state-managed program, and, through it, selected services are paid for that are different in each state. There are no incentives in the program for agencies to employ specific people, nor is it designed for the wealthy.

Comprehension/NA/Analysis

82. *Correct response: c*
The alternative answer choices are good things to consider and will promote quality and cost savings. However, answer choice **c** best defines the present national trend in financial restructuring of the health care delivery system.

Comprehension/Safe Care/
Implementation

83. *Correct response: c*
Answer choice **a** is an agency that combines an official and a proprietary agency together. It provides home care for a fee and public health services for no fee.

Answer choice **b** is free standing and established as a for-profit business.

Answer choice **d** provides mandated services and is not for profit.

Comprehension/NA/NA

84. *Correct response: b*
All home care services are ordered and directed by the physician. The other practitioners have responsibilities in carrying out parts of the services to the home care client.

Comprehension/NA/NA

85. *Correct response: b*
Physical therapists do not assist with personal care in the home. They do not supervise other caregivers or work so closely with other agencies.

Application/Safe Care/Implementation

86. *Correct response: d*
Answer choices **a, b,** and **c** are incorrect. Physical assessment skills, nursing care, and decision-making skills are important in both settings, but are needed more in the home care setting due to the autonomous nature of the practice.

Application/Safe Care/Implementation

87. *Correct response: c*
Home health nursing populations are older, have acute and chronic illnesses, and have home health nursing visits because they are ill or injured.

Application/Health Promotion/
Implementation

88. *Correct response: c*
Because this order is out of the normal range of doses for this medication, you should withhold the ordered dose until clarified by the physician. Checking with others, having family or caregivers follow up, or recommending the medication be taken and side effects watched for are dangerous practices that threaten the health, and perhaps the life, of the client while placing decisions in the hands of someone else, even nonprofessionals. You are the primary professional caregiver and need to follow up with the most restrictive approach to promote client safety.

Application/Safe Care/Implementation

89. *Correct response: c*
The incident report is completed and kept within the agency. Completion of this document is not mentioned in the client's chart, not placed in the chart, nor reserved for the client's lawyer. It is an internal document for quality and risk management. Data collected from

incident reports assist agencies in changing or reinforcing practices and protocols.

Application/Safe Care/Implementation

90. *Correct response: d*

Answer choices **a, b,** and **c** describe consolidation, integration, and segmentation, respectively, the three other modifications to agency internal structure.

Comprehension/Safe Care/Assessment

91. *Correct response: b*

Answer choice **a** better describes the Medicaid program.

In answer choice **c,** all home care services are directed by a physician, making physician care essential to home care services.

In answer choice **d,** social work services are covered under Medicare along with other services.

Comprehension/Safe Care/Assessment

92. *Correct response: a*

Alternative answer choices **b** and **c** are impossible to deliver with such a small staff and the distances needed to be traveled.

Answer choice **d** is not one of the considerations in organizational patterns of service.

Application/Safe Care/Implementation

93. *Correct response: c*

Answer choices **a** and **b** are the same and work better in suburban or rural settings.

Answer choice **d** is not one of the considerations in organizational patterns of service.

Application/Safe Care/Implementation

94. *Correct response: c*

Client outcomes are the measurable criteria of caregiving, and achieved outcomes are the goal of any quality management program. The other answer choices are important but are not the overall goal of a quality management program.

Analysis/Safe Care/Evaluation

95. *Correct response: b*

The alternative responses are normal occurrences during the prenatal period and alone do not signal a need for home health nursing services.

Comprehension/Safe Care/Analysis

96. *Correct response: d*

Handwashing is the most important infection control measure. Each of the alternative responses is important, but does not have the overall positive effect that handwashing does to control infection.

Comprehension/Safe Care/Analysis

97. *Correct response: b*

Client conditions identified in answer choices **a, c,** and **d** have been receiving care for many years by nurses in home health agencies.

Application/Safe Care/Implementation

98. *Correct response: b*

Answer choices **a, c,** and **d** are not true. Many agencies use nursing diagnoses. They do not hinder nursing care in any setting, nor is it mandatory that they be used.

Application/Safe Care/Planning

99. *Correct response: c*

None of the people mentioned in the alternative answer choices are the appropriate people to deliver the mentioned equipment. A durable medical equipment company delivers, sets up, and at times instructs in safe use.

Application/Safe Care/Implementation

100. *Correct response: c*

Technology has been a part of home health nursing for 20 years or more. Both home care and acute care nurses need to be familiar with technology. Technology is increasing in home care and will continue to do so.

Application/Safe Care/Implementation

Index

Page numbers followed by *f* indicate figures, by *d*, displays, and by *t*, tables.